Leave That Behind

Diet-Free Weight Loss
in 5 Simple Steps

by Linda K. Cobb

Cover Design by Cathi Stevenson
Editing by Maura Leon and Heather Taylor
Proofreading by Melody Masi
Interior Design by Rudy Milanovich

ISBN: 978-0-9716180-4-6

The Coaching Company, Inc.

Printed in the United States of America
First Printing, 2015

Dedication

This book is dedicated to you, the person who battles the discouragement of dieting to lose weight or maintain lost weight. In our culture that reveres thin bodies while promoting fast food on every corner, you must run a gauntlet of conflict every day. I want you to be free of the battle. May my story give you hope, and may the tools I've learned aid your journey. I am not special, but I am living proof that permanent change is possible—and is worth the effort.

Acknowledgments

So many people have influenced my journey, beginning with my brother, David, and my parents, Albert and Bernita Curtis. They pulled me through my darkest days and provided me with a lifelong spiritual foundation. And though they have all passed on, they continuously inspire me to offer my best.

Thanks also go to the childhood friends who teased me. Their words that defined my self-image long ago ultimately strengthened my resolve to prove them wrong.

My deepest gratitude goes to my husband, Ron, who has steadfastly believed in me and supported my life's work so unconditionally. His faith in me has been a great source of strength over the years, and his conscientious nature and self-sufficiency have freed me to pursue my goals.

Special thanks must also go to my dear friends, Valerie Holloway and Anne DuBois, for their unwavering support and encouragement to finally get this book written. I'm lucky to have such friends, who are not only talented professionals but also playmates and sounding boards. Without them, I would not have found my purpose nor rediscovered my fun self. Valerie and Anne, you have both enriched my life journey beyond measure.

I must also acknowledge Lisa Nasrallah, who is a shining example of friendship and fun-loving achievement. Thank you, Lisa, for introducing me to CrossFit and showing me that I'm capable of far more than I thought possible.

And my heartfelt appreciation goes to Kirstin, Susan, and Angie, my workout pals, who support me and help keep me committed to exercise.

My thanks also go to the group of friends and supporters who served as a focus group for this material. You provided valuable feedback and the encouragement that I needed to embark on this endeavor.

And finally, thanks to Keith and Maura Leon—book wizards, visionaries, and editors—who compiled my daunting collection of materials and personal stories, gave them order and continuity, and ultimately, got this book into print.

Contents

Introduction

WHY DIETS DON'T WORK

Are you tired of diets that focus on meal plans and exercise regimens?

If so, you're not alone. Just choosing a plan can be tedious. It is exhausting to generate the energy to stick to it day after day—especially in a culture that shows us a popular idea of the ideal body every day while it supersizes our meal portions and escalates our calorie consumption. It's no wonder there are problems with weight in our country today!

One in three adults in the United States is now overweight or obese.[1] Over one hundred million people go on a diet every year, and most of those dieters make three or four attempts. Every year, a new weight-loss method appears and lures you into believing that this diet plan will work. If you've ever felt defeated by that cycle, you're clearly not alone. It's a seductive promise, and every year, it generates huge profits for an entire industry.

People experience not only health problems but also guilt and shame over these added pounds. And that's why weight loss—an industry of diet companies, weight-loss supplement manufacturers, diet book authors, and obesity doctors—is big business.

In fact, MarketData Enterprises, a market research firm that has tracked diet products and programs since 1989, reports that the U.S. weight-loss market has grown from thirty billion in 1992 to a whopping sixty billion in 2014.[3] And yet, rates of obesity are rising every year, not just in the United States but globally. Obviously, the so-called solutions we're buying are not delivering the results we're so desperately seeking.

Why?

If your problem is solved, you'll stop buying the latest fad diet, book, pill, or fitness craze. And yet, all the methods that claim to be breakthroughs hide the truth: they still rely on a flawed model.

The traditional route to permanent weight loss has focused on changing your diet and adding exercise. That's what you've probably been told because that's what most health educators were taught (even as our culture was moving in the opposite direction.) There's nothing new or revealing about how traditional diet and exercise plans work; change your behavior (eat this, move that) and achieve results. Use self-discipline (aka *willpower*) to follow the plan, and you will reach your goal.

So if this isn't working, is it because you and one billion other people lack willpower?

Or is there something missing in this equation—something so fundamental that without it, no diet or exercise plan could possibly work?

What is willpower?

Isn't it necessary to have lots of it for any real change to occur?

The following three statements will give you some information concerning the validity of willpower as it relates to dieting.

1. A study published in The *Journal of the American Medical Association* in 2005 found that regardless of the diet attempted (Weight Watchers, Atkins, Paleo, and Ornish), 25 percent of patients lost an average of 5 percent of their baseline weight after one year, and 10 percent of patients lost an average of 10 percent. Dropout rates from the study were more than 40 percent. Doctors conducting the study found that *poor sustainability and adherence rates* resulted in modest weight loss.[4]
2. Dr. Michael R. Lowe, a professor of clinical psychology at the MCP Hahnemann University in Philadelphia, said that he and others viewed willpower as *"essentially, an explanatory fiction."* Saying that someone lacks willpower

"leaves people with the sense they understand why the behavior occurred when in reality, all they've done is label the behavior, not explain it," he said.[5]

3. *"There is no magical stuff inside of you called willpower* that should somehow override nature," said Dr. James C. Rosen, a professor of psychology at the University of Vermont. *"It's a metaphor* that most chronically overweight dieters buy into."[6]

These three references indicate that there is no such thing as willpower, or "sustainability and adherence," as the first group put it. Frankly, I find that quite a relief. For the longest time, I thought my lack of willpower was some kind of birth defect. Rest assured that you weren't born with it either, and you don't need it.

If there is no such thing as willpower, then why can't we stick with it?

What causes us to fail, time and again, on diets?

We fail because we've been sold an incomplete formula—a formula that in fact, ensures our failure.

Why?

Often, it's because well-meaning health educators are simply passing along what they've been taught. Unintentionally, they omit an essential element because it wasn't part of their training. However in the last twenty years, diet programs have grown to become a very significant business—a business that wants your dollars.

And here's something that should really make you angry:

Businesses that sell diet programs are built on repeat business.

They know that if you are constantly dissatisfied with your results, you will continue to be in pain, and you will continue to seek relief. That means you'll continue to buy anything that promises to produce the result you desire. So it's not really intended to help you get past the problem. It's intended to keep you hooked into the problem. That makes me really angry, and I hope it makes you angry too. I hope you want to be free of the whole weight issue, and I want to share with you everything I know about how to do that.

Now, I don't believe there's a knowledge deficit about food and exercise. Any healthy eating and exercise program has the potential to work. If you burn off more than you take in, your weight will decrease. But the truth is that *you don't need to be on a diet*.

Most of us have a pretty good idea of what we should be eating, and we know that we should exercise.

Would you say that's true?

If so, then what's the problem?

Why do we all struggle with weight so much?

Consider this: If there is no such thing as willpower, then **perhaps diets don't work because you haven't changed your thinking**. Perhaps that is what will make you change your habits permanently.

I've watched the diet industry my whole adult life, and it makes me crazy that no one is addressing how to think differently to lose and maintain weight. We're one of the richest countries in the world. We have the means to educate masses of people, and yet so many struggle needlessly.

Without that missing link, people stay stuck and unhappy. That's why they get hooked by the promise of each new diet program. I know, because I was that person. I want you to know that there's a better way — a permanent way.

If you're unhealthy because of your behavior, and you can't change your behavior with willpower, then aren't you glad that you *can* change it with your thinking?

Behaviors are the actions resulting from thoughts. Change your thoughts and beliefs, and the behaviors will line up to match them. The traditional model of dieting is flawed because it does not address the thinking that creates the behavior in the first place. To change your behavior, you must change your thinking. (I'll cover this concept in much more detail later.)

Traditional Dieting

1. You learn new BEHAVIORS.
2. You try to apply WILLPOWER.
3. You get poor RESULTS.

Permanent Health

1. You change your THINKING.
2. Your BEHAVIOR changes.
3. You get good RESULTS.

The good news is that lots of people have successfully gone on a diet and lost weight permanently.

Why do some people have success on diets?

Have they all changed the way they think?

Yes!

For any real and permanent change to take place, they had to change their behavior. To do that for the long term, they had to change their thinking.

HOW TO CREATE POSITIVE CHANGE

The principles of success are actually well known now. They are not a quick fix; they require effort. Rather than being a list of how-to's, they are more like laws. Just as gravity is accepted as a law of physics, there are natural laws that govern the results you create in your life. Understand those laws and live in harmony with them, and you can create your best life, no matter where your life is currently.

Most self-help books attempt to show you how to fix yourself or your life. This presumes that something about you needs fixing. If you're like me and have read lots of self-help books, you may have consistently reinforced the internal message that you are somehow broken. When that's your focus, you'll always find something (i.e., when you're a hammer, everything looks like a nail), so you'll always need more self-help books.

As a coach, I want so much more for you. I want you to create the life you truly desire, not just fix your current life, so you can tolerate it.

What if you're not broken?

What if all the answers you ever needed are already inside you, and all you need is a way to tap into the inner knowing that you already possess?

What if it isn't really new knowledge you need at all, but just a way to remember what your core self has always known?

That's what I want to share with you. It's a process that will not only give you the results you want in your physical body, but you can use it for your whole life—anywhere, anytime, for any area of your life. As you practice the process over time, you'll find that it will eliminate the need for advice from others. You'll learn to trust what we might call your inner guide.

There is really only one thing you need to do: feel good.

As you read this book, keep in mind that as human beings, we are more alike than we are different. Throughout our lives, we all have two characteristics in common:

1. Change
2. Choice

We will all experience change, and we all have the power of choice. Because we have a conscious mind, we all have the ability to choose our responses.

Yes, you have that ability.

It may not feel like it right now, but you can change your responses just like I learned to do. And when you do that consistently over time, you create the changes you've always wanted. It's a simple process, but it's not easy because it will require you to trust the process.

That's how you can succeed, and it's what this book is all about. By consciously deciding to change and using the power of your mind, you can install practices that will remove all the guesswork and will ensure success every time.

When you change how you think, everything changes.

To support you in your process, this book contains two things:

1. The story of my own personal journey from overweight, unfulfilled, and suicidal to happy, healthy, and successful.
2. A structured program to expand your awareness, with practices aimed at creating well-being through a healthy mind, body, and spirit as the result of deliberate choice.

Components include five chapters about my personal journey, along with five steps to your success. The steps need not be done in order, nor must any one of them be completed prior to moving on to the next step. The objective of this program is to give you a structure with which to apply the universal laws of success.

To get the most benefit from this new journey, keep a journal or notebook handy, and write your answers to the questions posed in this book. This will help you to clarify your intentions and will also provide you with a document to review over time.

For most of our lives, we were taught to use correct behaviors. Few of us learned how to effectively use the power of our minds, and fewer still learned how to access our inner wisdom. Yet it's this inner wisdom that is at the heart of all the good we have ever created.

You will be learning new skills, practicing the skills to link your mind and your spirit, and developing unshakable faith in yourself by noticing the outcomes you create. As you make this commitment to being your best self, track how the universe responds, and savor your milestones along the way.

Our greatest teachers have taught us that we can achieve whatever we set our minds to. The greatest coaches have helped people out-perform their former records. The elements of success are known but not widely practiced. These principles are not new but tried and true. When we understand the principles and apply them consistently, we all have the ability to create successful results. That is my sincere promise to you.

On this journey, your highest priority must be to connect with your inner wisdom, for that is your most accurate compass.

Notes

1. Cynthia L. Ogden, Margaret D. Carroll, Brian K. Kit, and Katherine M. Flegal, "Prevalence of Childhood and Adult Obesity in the United States, 2011–2012," Journal of the American Medical Association 311, no. 8 (2014): 806–814, doi:10.1001/jama.2014.732.

2. MarketData Enterprises, Inc., "The U.S. Weight Loss Market: 2014 Status Report and Forecast" (February, 2015).
3. Catey Hill, "10 Things the Weight Loss Industry Won't Tell You," MarketWatch (January 14, 2014), http://www.marketwatch.com/story/10-things-the-weight-loss-industry-wont-tell-you-2014-01-10.
4. Michael L. Dansinger, Joi Augustin Gleason, John L. Griffith, et al., "Comparison of the Atkins, Ornish, Weight Watchers, and Zone Diets for Weight Loss and Heart Disease Risk Reduction," Journal of the American Medical Association 293 no. 1 (January 5, 2005): 43–53, doi:10.1001/jama.293.1.43.
5. Jane Fritsch, "Scientists Unmask Diet Myth: Willpower," New York Times (October 5, 1999), http://www.nytimes.com/1999/10/05/health/scientists-unmask-diet-myth-willpower.html.
6. Ibid.

Other:

Bradley C. Johnston, Steve Kanters, Kristofer Bandayrel, et al., "Comparison of Weight Loss Among Named Diet Programs in Overweight and Obese Adults," JAMA 312, no. 9 (September 3, 2014), doi:10.1001/jama.2014.10397.

Summary: The weight-loss differences between individual named diets were small with likely little importance to those seeking weight loss. This supports the practice of recommending any diet that a patient will adhere to in order to lose weight.

Chapter One

From Desperation to Discovery

I've been studying this phenomenon called *success* for most of my life. It's a passion of mine, borne out of my frustration to lose weight. I used to try every diet that came along and then get depressed when I didn't make any progress. In fact, I often gained weight on a diet.

Has that ever happened to you?

I had two loving, responsible parents, but I especially adored my dad. So when I was four years old and he said, "you must always think of others first," I believed him. I'm sure that I had been selfish about something, and it was an appropriate lesson for me. Neither one of us knew then that my young mind installed that message as an absolute.

Of course, it wasn't my father's intention, but from that day forward, I always thought about other people first. I became adept at knowing what others needed and how I could please them. Eventually, I developed low self-esteem as I became increasingly blind to my own needs and desires.

I also became hypersensitive to others. It became almost intolerable if I felt that I'd hurt another person or even inconvenienced them. It upset me greatly when at eight years old, I was riding my bike and accidentally knocked something out of another kid's hand as I rode past him. He got very angry, and I cried all night about my blunder. Just the thought that I had upset someone was something I couldn't bear.

This hypersensitivity may have developed my capacities for empathy and intuition (which did help me, years later, as a counselor). But as a kid, it hampered my self-awareness. In elementary school, I began making choices based on what I perceived other people wanted and how I thought that they perceived me.

I was heavy growing up, and I was tall for my age. In fact, I had the distinction of being the tallest person in my elementary school. Plus, I had red hair, crooked teeth, and glasses. I wanted desperately to fit in, but I felt perpetually odd. In order to protect myself from being teased, I became self-conscious and increasingly shy.

My story is not remarkable. Heck, lots of us were awkward and self-conscious when we were kids. Those cruel kid comments began forming my self-image, as they do for many of us.

Larry in fourth grade laughed and said, "Look! Linda has a little head and a great big body."

I was mortified. I went home from school and ate cookies to console myself.

In sixth grade, when I discovered boys, I liked whoever was the tallest even though I was still always larger. My size began to drive my choices pretty early in life. I did have friends — soon, I even had a boyfriend — but I didn't feel good about my body or myself.

I wasn't an unhappy kid, but I was very insecure. More than anything, I wanted to feel good in my body and not feel self-conscious.

I remember praying: *Please, God, let me just have blond hair and blue eyes and be five-foot-two and petite.*

Of course, I had already surpassed five-foot-two, but I longed to be like the ones who were known as pretty girls. Feeling trapped and self-conscious in my big body, I limited myself to a small circle of close friends and rarely participated in group games, even at recess. I played no organized sports, but I loved to ride my bicycle. I did try some physical activities, but I would always make sure that my friends wouldn't see me; I would only allow my parents or my family to see me. I tried synchronized swimming and other things that I really enjoyed doing — even dance classes, which I still love to do.

I consoled myself with food. After-school snacks became a normal and much-anticipated reward for me. I felt hungry all the time.

Because I couldn't seem to have just one of anything, Mom would say, "Moderation, Linny, moderation."

Moderation?

I remember thinking: *How do people do that?*

The thought of eating one cookie just never crossed my mind. Being regularly reminded about moderation, I eventually thought of myself as someone who wasn't capable of it.

I began to sneak things to eat or stop at the candy store on my way home, so my mom wouldn't see it. By the time I was eleven years old, that had became a regular routine. That's when I became addicted to candy. Once I started, I wouldn't stop eating it until it was all gone.

It was no surprise that I got heavier. By the time I entered junior high school, I was definitely overweight. My self-consciousness increased along with my negative body image. Once again, I isolated myself and consoled myself with food.

Even as a young child, I recall people commenting about my mother's beauty. As I grew up, I could see what they meant, and I had such admiration for her. Unfortunately, I began to compare myself to her, which gave me another reason to feel badly about myself. She *never* overate. To me, she seemed completely in control and moderate all the time. By contrast, I felt completely out of control. I didn't know how she maintained such discipline. I ate to feel better and probably to avoid the impossible effort of trying to be like her.

I wanted to be invisible, so I hid behind the shield of shyness, afraid of anything that would call attention to me.

I remember a well-meaning aunt saying, "Linda, you just have big bones."

Her message acknowledged my misery and was intended to help me feel better, and for a while, it did. In fact, I used that phrase as an excuse for so long that I almost believed it.

I just have big bones.

Unfortunately, that didn't make me feel better in my body. (I later learned that I don't have big bones at all. I actually have a rather small frame.)

By the time I graduated from the ninth grade, my best friend, Jane, had mortified me by nicknaming me Lardo. She dubbed me that because, on a double-date mishap, I had gotten into the back seat of the car and split my pants wide open! Her nickname for me stuck with her, and the shame stuck with me. We actually remained friends, but the hurt also remained. Perhaps I was simply too insecure to consider losing a friend.

That's when I began truly struggling with my weight. I wore a full girdle to try to look slimmer. What torture! I did anything I could to feel more like the girl that I wanted so badly to be. And I felt like an imposter the whole time.

In high school, I got heavier—and more desperate to fit in. That's when I started dieting. I failed on every diet I tried, which reinforced my low self-esteem. I read about what people called *willpower* and eventually concluded that everybody else must be born with it. I must have had some kind of birth defect because I just didn't have it. Of course, my increasingly low self-esteem plus little physical activity added up to even more pounds.

I go back to high school reunions now, and classmates say, "Gosh, I always thought you were so quiet and shy."

And I say to them, "Yeah, because you probably taunted me in grade school!"

I remember making a very strong decision that college was going to be different and that I was going to lose weight. At that point, I did lose about fifteen pounds. That was out of sheer determination, every single day, doing the same thing. I began exercising for the first time in my life.

It was a short-term goal, however, because I decided: *That's what I'm going to do for this period of time because there is no way I'm going to college that heavy.*

I had some success, and it was thrilling! It really was the thing that allowed me to suddenly become adventurous and go away to college. Fear fueled me too.

I had heard plenty of messages like:

"When you go to college, you're going to gain twenty pounds."

"Watch out for the *freshman fifteen*."

By the time I got to college, I was terrified that I'd gain the weight back. So I learned how to starve myself. I did get thin, but of course, I also got unhealthy.

I quit having periods.

My hair started falling out.

I was tired all the time.

I came home from college on winter break and shocked my parents, who marched me right to the doctor.

Our family doctor said, "Linda, you need to start eating."

After doing that, I gained back all that weight plus twenty pounds more. I was miserable.

When I went back to college, I resumed dieting and stopped eating again. That led to lots of yo-yo dieting, which just made me feel crazy. What I wanted—more than life itself—was to wear jeans with the pockets close together in the back. At nineteen, that was the image I longed to become.

Of course, what I really wanted was freedom. I wanted to go anywhere, do anything, and wear anything I wanted without feeling like my body was holding me back.

I was so tired of the whole thing, and I wanted freedom from having to feel like I had to deal with it all the time. But each time my weight fluctuated, I got more depressed.

Eventually, I got so depressed that I decided to kill myself. I made a plan to do it. At the time, I lived on the top floor of a twelve-story dormitory. I would just open the window and throw myself onto the parking lot below. That was my plan.

On a particularly desperate night, I climbed onto the big frame of the opened window and stood poised to jump.

Then, a little voice in my head said, very clearly:

Linda, that would be a really weenie thing to do.

I wish it was something more profound and poetic, but that's what the voice said. In other words, something from deep inside was calling me a coward.

That got my attention, and then, very quickly, I got another strong message:

Killing yourself would deeply hurt your family.

I stopped and thought about them. I could kill myself, but I couldn't intentionally hurt them. I managed to get myself out of the window frame and back into my room, where I collapsed on the floor, crying uncontrollably.

By the time I stopped crying, I felt completely exhausted and utterly hopeless. I had no clue what to do. But in that moment, I made two very important decisions.

1. I decided to live — even if it was only for the sake of not hurting my parents.
2. I decided that somehow, I was going to get past the whole issue of weight and finally be free. I didn't know how I was going to do it, but I knew that I was going to have what I wanted, which was to never again let weight rule my life.

The next day, I kept thinking about the voice in my head that had called me a coward. I thought it was supposed to love me, but it really made me angry. (I now realize that it was that anger that gave me the energy to change the direction of my life. Perhaps the voice did love me.)

As I looked around my room, I saw piles of diet books. I realized that I had been relying on the advice of all the people who wrote those books, and it hadn't worked for me.

I said to myself: *Either I'm so incredibly special that diets work for everybody else and just not for me, or it's all a big, fat lie!*

None of these diet books were helping me get past this problem.

Why couldn't I stick with any of them?

Every new diet book promised to make me thinner, sexier, or happier, and each one was going to do it faster than the last one. Each one offered the one thing that I was so desperate for: hope.

Then, it finally sunk in; they *were* lying to me. The authors knew what I was desperate for, and they sold me what I needed. At that point—probably for the first time in my life—I got really, *really* angry. I realized that if I was ever going to get past this, I was going to have to figure it out for myself.

As I threw all of my diet books in the dumpster, I thought: *Something is missing here.*

And then, I did something I had never done before.

I changed the question.

Up until that point, my question had always been:

How do I lose weight?

I now asked myself:

What creates success?

How do successful people achieve their goals?

I went to the library and began reading biographies of people I admired, like the Wright brothers, Helen Keller, and Benjamin Franklin. What I learned fascinated me. Although their stories varied greatly, I began to notice that there were some elegantly simple common threads that successful people all used to create goals—that they all did basically the same things to achieve results:

They clearly decided what they wanted, and then they acted as if they had their goal before they had it.

Although their lives were often very difficult, they were absolutely committed to something larger than themselves, and they stayed focused on that commitment until they achieved their purpose. None of the stories made that look easy, but the principles they applied were fundamentally quite simple. And most importantly, they did not rely on the advice of others; they all created their own paths.

After studying dozens of books, I ended up thinking: *Wow, can it really be that simple?*

Then, I started doing what they did.

I kept reminding myself that the old way wasn't working and that I was just going to try out this new way. I made a commitment to follow this path instead.

I began, slowly and incrementally, to trust in myself and not rely on diet books. I kept being tempted by them because I really wanted a quick solution out of my desperation. But I kept reminding myself that they didn't work for me.

While I'd love to tell you that everything in my life fell into place and was set to music at that point, it was not at all that simple. In fact, I spent the next ten years struggling to make those concepts work for me. I did, however, manage to stabilize enough so I could finish college and have a social life.

In those days, there weren't really any books about the mechanics of creating success. So even though I'd thrown away my diet books and had a few new ideas, I didn't realize yet that I'd have to blaze my own trail. I'd been taught to follow the advice of experts, and I'd learned from so-called diet experts that I should focus on this thing called weight and get rid of it.

Well, when you're on a diet, what do you think about?

It's either food or weight, right?

What I learned was that successful people focus on what they want, not what they don't want. That's a very big difference. In order to act as if you have something that you want, you must first identify what you want. Then, you must focus on that.

I remember forgiving myself, periodically.

I would buy a diet magazine here and there, and then I would realize: *Oh yeah, I forgot. I'm not going to do it that way.*

I had to keep reinforcing that commitment.

I learned how to focus on what I wanted rather than what I didn't want. I allowed myself the freedom to pretend — to act as if I had already achieved my goal. I stopped comparing the inside of me to the outside of others, which is what I realized I had been doing. I stopped letting approval from others rule my life.

It really was a progression.

It went from comparing myself to others, having low self-esteem and a poor self-image, having a desperate desire to fit in, and trying many things to the turning point of making that decision to live and to find a new way, letting myself get angry when I realized that I had been betrayed by the very people I had expected to be experts, and finding a whole new approach.

That was the progression of how I overcame my obstacles. It wasn't a quick or an easy process because I hadn't yet found any books on how to be successful. I was strictly going by what I thought successful people did.

Using this process, I created my commitment to seek tools that I could use, at first, just to get me through the day and then, throughout my life. I use many of those tools to this day, and I keep adding to my tools all the time. My original commitment — something I wanted more than life itself — was to wear blue jeans with the pockets close together. Over time, as my commitment has expanded and even changed, I have always found that the more my reason includes others, the more solid it is.

Here I am all these years later, and I have managed to keep off forty pounds for the last thirty years.

Step One:
Set Your Intention

Once you test it for yourself, you'll find that this process will consistently guide you to positive outcomes. It can be used to remedy current issues as well as to create a roadmap for a richly fulfilling future.

CLARITY

Commitment is the first step toward deliberately creating change. We live in a culture that reveres thinness while it feeds us food that makes us fat. It takes real commitment to stay healthy.

When you create an intention to "be healthy," "lose weight," or "increase energy levels," there is generally more to what you want than just those words. Asking yourself what you really want will accelerate the process by helping you to clarify your intention and narrow your focus.

Notice Your Feelings

No matter where you begin, be as clear as you can be. You may find that you come back and modify your wants and your whys as you move through the process.

The best indicator for knowing if your answers are really in line with what you want is how you feel. If your answers feel good (i.e., your energy goes up), then you are on the right track. Your feelings will be your strongest indicator because, *when you feel good, you are actually getting closer to what you want.*

Ask Yourself Questions

Have you clearly identified the deepest intentions you hold for your life?

Ask yourself:

If I weren't struggling with my weight, where would my focus be?

What do I really want?

What is my highest intention?

Why do I want that?

When I have that, how will my life be different?

How do I feel when I think about having what I want?

Determine Your Viewpoint

Establish your deepest *why*. Whether you approach it from a positive viewpoint or a negative one, just go as deep as you can.

For example:

A positive intention is...

I intend to enjoy living in my body.

A negative intention is...

I intend to never again allow my body to restrict my freedom.

...or...

I will never again allow my body to restrict my freedom to go anywhere, do anything, or wear whatever I want.

While people vary in which approach helps them initially, establishing the highest positive intention is what creates a healthy life.

The Difference Between Intentions and Goals

When you are committed to a clear intention, you're less likely to be seduced by short-term goals. While short-term goals like "lose twenty pounds for the wedding" don't create lasting results, they can be used to kick-start your progress. A short-term goal with a clear long-term intention works like starter fluid; it can build belief quickly, so you feel enough confidence to keep moving forward.

Setting intentions is not the same as making goals. Goal-making is a valuable skill. It involves envisioning a future outcome, then planning, applying discipline, and working hard to achieve it. Goals help provide direction to your life. With goals, the future is always the focus. Goals are not concerned with what is happening to you in the present moment.

Setting an intention is quite different. Intentions are not oriented toward a future outcome. Instead, they are a practice that is focused on how you are *being* in the present moment. Your attention is on the ever-present *now* in the constantly changing flow of life. You set your intentions based on understanding what matters most to you. When you set an intention, you make a commitment to align your actions with your inner values.

Intentions guide the present while goals guide the future. Goals are limited by a defined end result, so they don't generally become part of our beliefs or boundaries. For that reason, goals are often much easier to abandon and are best utilized for short-term results along the path of your broader intentions.

Figure 1. Intentions and Goals

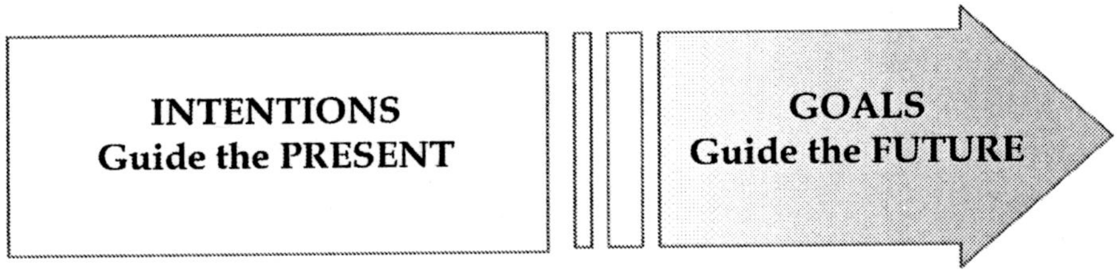

An intention is a *presupposition*; it's something that is believed before it's manifested. As such, it creates a powerful imprint that can guide your behavior in the present moment. Intentions direct your mind toward a desired outcome. When you create intentions that are linked with your core desires, you line up scattered energy and focus it powerfully in one direction.

Intentions are a practice, not an outcome or destination. You don't just set intentions and then forget about them; you live them, moment by moment, every day. Goals can provide direction and help you be a more effective person. But being grounded in intention is what provides integrity and unity in your life. It allows you to maintain momentum and not get too attached to narrow outcomes.

Strong intentions also have the power to reprogram and expand limiting subconscious boundaries. "I intend to be healthy" is a perfect example. I want you to make an intention to be healthy right now. And part of making that intention means you are living in the present moment and accepting what is.

CHOICE

If you would like to convert the negative aspects of your life to positive, you must make different choices.

Do you know how to change how you make choices?

There is a science to self-development, and the good news is that it contains predictable elements that we can all learn. The only difference between success and failure is your decision to apply the elements.

Your Power to Create

You have at your disposal the common traits available to all humans. You will forever experience change, which means that you are never stuck in one place for long. And you have the power to choose. In fact, that is how you created the life you currently live.

Unfortunately, most of us were not taught how results are actually created. So forgive yourself. You couldn't have known. Sadly, "how to create a successful life" has not been taught in traditional schools. So you made choices that, with time and repetition, created beliefs, behaviors, and habits that, in turn, created your life.

If you look at your life, you will see how your choices manifested.

- Those things in your life that you love, you created.
- Those things in your life that you dislike, you created.

That may not seem like good news, but it is. It means that you have the power to recreate your life. It doesn't matter what your choices have been in the past. Right now, you can make informed choices, based on what you want most in your life, and over time, those choices will ensure that you create the life you truly desire. Learn how results are created, and you'll forever grow through all the changes of life.

Directing Your Energy

Life can be difficult, but it is not random. Things do happen for a reason. The reason is energy — your own, along with the energy in your environment. While energy appears in many forms, its properties are predictable. Energy contains movement. It's constantly changing, and it can be converted but not destroyed. Learn to direct your own energy, and you'll know how to recreate any aspect of your life.

Think about your body and all its miraculous functions.

- Your cells are in motion, even at rest, and are constantly changing as you move through time.
- Your digestive system converts food into energy.
- Your intellectual and physical efforts convert labor into money.
- Your thoughts convert ideas into behaviors.

In fact, your whole life is about change and energy conversion.

How will you choose to direct your energy?

Do life's changes energize you with possibilities or fatigue you with distractions?

If you'd like to enjoy a richly satisfying life, you can learn to direct this energy to create your own positive changes.

Since everything contains energy and interacts with your own energy in some way, the only question is: How will it interact?

The answer to that is within your control. It's entirely up to you.

As a human being, you have a built-in energy-converting ability, and you can access it to help you create success in any area of your life. It will illuminate your path and speed your progress. It's actually a simple process, based on science and years of experience, but it's not easy.

If you have ever tried to simply change your behavior, then you probably know that it rarely works and doesn't last. To truly create what you desire most and create it in the most efficient way, you must understand your own energy and the energy around you, and you must know how to use the natural laws that create outcomes. You must understand how you get what you get. Equipped with this knowledge, you can consistently make good choices that are right for you. Those choices will, in turn, create a life that fulfills you.

TRUST

The principles in this book will empower you to harness your energy and direct it toward positive change. They will expand your awareness, structure your practice, and ensure positive results.

Oddly, the most difficult part is this: *You must trust the process.*

Thinking Differently

Change does require energy. And generating sufficient energy requires your focused attention. But it may surprise you to know that *your focused thought is the critical element for creating change.*

Are you willing to practice thinking differently in order to create positive change in your life?

To move forward and efficiently create successful outcomes will require daily practice that will often involve going against your own thoughts (as you currently experience them). Once you test it for yourself, however, you'll find that this process will consistently guide you to positive outcomes. It can be used to remedy current issues as well as to create a roadmap for a richly fulfilling future.

Chapter Two

Whose Life is This?

Once I learned to change the question (from *How can I lose weight?* to *What creates success?*), I realized that I was not broken. My mind naturally found the questions I needed to ask myself. Gradually, I began to feel a little bit better. That helped me to focus more on college. It helped me get past my inhibitions and meet people again. (I had become very isolated in my depression, something that, at the time, I didn't realize I had.) For the first time in my life, I felt more comfortable in my body. This boosted my confidence, and I was willing to try new things, like becoming an exchange student in Switzerland and a camp counselor at a theater arts camp.

Even though I felt more comfortable in my body, I did not feel secure about my body. A lot of my thoughts were driven by always being hyper-aware of every little thing that I ate. While I did manage to keep my weight down for a while, it was a struggle.

Eventually, I met a man and fell in love—at least, to the degree that I was able to understand love at the age of twenty-two. If there was one thing I knew about this man it was that he would be successful. I don't think I defined it quite like that, but I had a very strong belief that he was someone who would be successful.

Soon after college, we got married. As our marriage developed, we did a lot of traveling. We actually moved twelve times in twelve years, and I got to experience a lot of great things. Because of my husband's business, we lived in ski towns for many years, made lots of money, and had a very exciting life.

On the outside, life looked really good.

As my husband's career skyrocketed, I followed his star. While that felt very exciting for many years, what I didn't realize while we were living this life was that the more successful he got, the worse I felt. My self-esteem was actually going lower as his was going higher, creating a very big gulf between us.

I did enjoy skiing if I could do it by myself or perhaps with my husband, but when I was with a social group of people, I got very insecure. I felt like I was around all of these beautiful people, and even though on the outside I may have looked like I fit in, on the inside I felt like an impostor. It was a very stressful time for me because I felt on the verge of being out of control — like I was just barely hanging on — nearly all the time.

I was using the one tool I had learned, which was to act as if I was successful. For a long time, it helped me, but I reached a point when acting-as-if wasn't making me feel good anymore. The more successful my husband became, the unhappier I became.

Once we decided to leave the ski towns and moved down out of the mountains into Boulder, I realized that I needed my own work. Because I had struggled with my weight for so long, I looked into buying a weight management franchise. This got me very excited.

I thought: *Here's a way that I can learn, keep myself aware, and also do something that's meaningful to me.*

My husband and I talked about it, and I made the purchase. This was the first time I had ever felt really proud of something that I had done. While that did help me, I soon learned the franchise's true concept.

At a training conference, the owner of the business said, "You need to understand that this company is built on repeat business."

That made me intensely angry. That was not at all why I had gotten into the business. I had gotten into it to save myself and to give myself a meaningful path to help others.

Because I didn't agree with their philosophy, I knew that I could not stay in that business, but I was very reluctant to leave. With my weight management franchise, I was able to focus on others. I felt useful, and I was getting validated. People were grateful to me, and I had been starving for that.

The reality was that I was a lousy businessperson. I managed to sell my franchise and break even, but I was left, once again, with no direction.

So I returned to work in our sports marketing company, among the beautiful people. I didn't even realize that the whole time I was among those people, I was focused on myself. The truth is that I treated them like objects. Of course, I wouldn't have said that at the time. In fact, I probably would have said that they treated *me* that way. That's how self-absorbed I was.

When I went back into sports marketing, I no longer had anyone telling me that I was doing a good job. I didn't have the validation, I didn't like the work, and to make matters worse, I was put in charge of handling the funds coming into our accounts, which gave me access to large amounts of money. I ended up coping with my unhappiness by using cocaine, which was very plentiful and available to me, especially with my ready access to cash.

The beauty of drugs and alcohol is that they make you feel more confident, which is what I came to rely on a great deal. The combination of those two substances enabled me to cope in a realm in which I still didn't feel like I belonged. I continued being extremely self-absorbed, hating my job, just getting through each day, and not having any better ideas. I wasn't a planner, so I had no plan; I was just responding to what happened in my life.

I knew that the drug wasn't good for me, but it helped me to feel better, get through the day, and keep up with a life that felt less and less like it was mine. Because my husband was very against cocaine use, I isolated myself and did it all in secret, so he wouldn't find out. Eventually, however, he did find out, and he got very, very angry.

In the interim, because I knew I was living in a way that I couldn't sustain, I had actually done some research on treatment options. I remembered a place I had come across—a Seventh-Day Adventist commune up in the mountains of Colorado—that had programs to lose weight and to stop smoking. When everything blew up, I called to find out if they would help me.

"Would you consider taking someone in and helping them get off of drugs? Have you ever taken people like that?"

"No, we haven't."

"Would you like to try?"

"Of course!"

So I arranged a day that I would go up there and begin their program.

I told them, "Just put me through whatever program you have, and I'll teach you about people with drug problems because you're missing a whole market."

I packed a little suitcase, and my husband drove me there. He wrote them a check, and he dropped me off at the end of a *very* long dirt road. I remember walking down that road, crying, carrying my little suitcase...and then, being welcomed with open arms.

During the program, I lived in a little house with a nurse and a couple of other people. We were totally cut off from the outside world, and I loved that. I felt like I was in my element.

Suddenly, I was not known as anything but Linda, and it didn't matter what I had done or where I was from. I was just a person who was there to work in the garden, go on long walks, do hot and cold therapies (hot steam baths and ice cold showers, very old-time remedies) and get healthy.

I felt totally accepted. We had church services, I sang in the choir, and I rediscovered things about myself. I felt very robust and healthy — healthier than I had felt in a long time.

Unfortunately, there was no after-care program, and when I tried to to re-enter my life, I really stumbled.

Upon returning home from the commune, I found that my husband, who traveled a great deal, wasn't there. He was out at the Los Angeles Olympics.

I thought to myself: *This is a good thing. I'll have some time to adjust.*

But when he called and said, "Linda, I want you to come out. Take the next plane, and come on out here with me," I went.

It was a very knee-jerk response.

I remember getting on that plane and having a little panic attack.

Oh, my gosh!

What am I doing?

I'm not ready.

Since I still had all my supply connections, when I landed, I called somebody and got some drugs to help me handle the situation.

At that point, an interesting thing happened.

The drugs didn't work.

I remember going into a bathroom, looking at myself in a mirror, and saying: *Now what are you going to do?*

Then, I thought: *Well, they weren't good drugs. I'll just buy some more.*

I did, and those didn't work either.

I was at yet another crossroads, and I realized: *They're just not working for me anymore. I'm going to have to actually figure out how to live my life.*

The life that I had created for twelve years no longer fit who I was, and even the drugs didn't compensate anymore. I was going to have to make a change. I would need to leave my life, or I was going to self-destruct. That felt like my only remaining choice.

At first, my newfound insights created confusion. My husband and I briefly tried counseling but ultimately agreed to discontinue the effort. Separation seemed like the only viable choice. At the same time, we were still good friends and were very reluctant to call it quits. We'd accomplished so much together, and we were now living in our fifth from-the-ground-up remodeled house.

That's a lot of sweat equity!

This was the house that we were supposed to live in for many years. Plus, we'd started three businesses, and our current sports marketing business was booming. But I knew that something had to change, and moving out of my house seemed like the easiest option since we'd recently purchased a small apartment building near the local university.

I thought:

I'll move into an apartment there.

I'll make a fresh start in new surroundings.

I can't possibly create my own life while I'm living under my husband's shadow.

I was desperate and confused, yet at the same time, excited about the prospect of having my own place. I figured that I could easily manage the apartments while working at another job.

I painted my new manager's apartment, set a date to move, lined up friends to help me, and rejoiced in my feeling of independence. I moved in and reveled in my darling garden-level apartment with the bright red pipes lining the ceiling.

This was freedom!

Even though I had no plan, for the first time in years, I was optimistic. I got a job as the administrative assistant to the president at our local hospital.

I was thrilled!

Having been raised by a hospital president, I felt right at home in that environment. While it took some time to adjust to the structure of a full-time job, the feelings of purpose and belonging were a welcome change.

Soon, I moved into another job, in the hospital's health education department, which was a great fit. Around the same time, I came to the realization that managing an apartment building full of college students was proving to be more than I could handle. After falling for yet another sad "can't pay the rent" story, I actively pursued a rental spot in the hospital's housing. My new boss pulled some strings, and almost immediately, I moved into a tiny cottage on the hospital grounds.

I thought: *This is the life I really want!*

Then, right after I had moved into the hospital cottage, they eliminated my job. Suddenly, I was jobless and was going to lose my housing. I scurried around and got another job, doing medical transcription for the speech pathology department.

Because of the environment and the team that I was a part of, I felt very comfortable. Even though I hated the work, I hated punching a time card, and I didn't make much money, I lived right across the street, and I felt very cared for. I ate my meals at the hospital, and I didn't have to worry about maintenance or repairs since they provided my housing. It was such a wonderful little cocoon. If things had gone differently, I probably would have stayed there for years.

Step Two:
Expand Your Awareness

"We are what we repeatedly do. Excellence, then, is not an act but a habit." ~Aristotle

THE CHANGE CYCLE

If you want to make changes in your life, it's important to understand the nature of change. All humans have change in common. We all go through change in our lives.

We change from:

- Babies into toddlers
- Toddlers into children
- Children into adults

These are changes over which we have no control.

Other times, we enter into change purposely.

- We decide to get married.
- We go to college.
- We get a job.

These are big changes in a person's life that are entered into, we hope, with excitement and anticipation.

Other changes, like the death of a loved one and the grief that follows, might be unexpected.

But whether change is embraced willingly or fraught with resistance, it goes through a predictable cycle that can be divided into three stages.

Figure 2. The Change Cycle

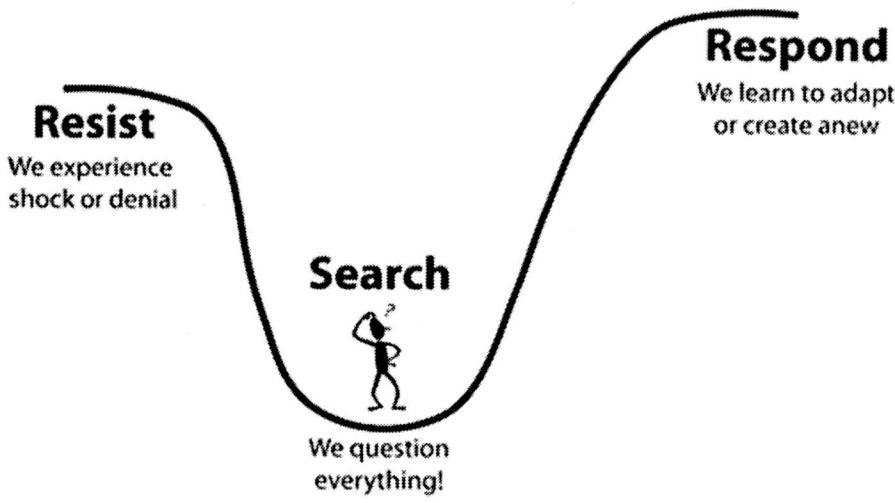

Recall the last time you experienced a change that was not your idea.

Initially, you probably resisted and didn't want to adapt because, even if you weren't happy before the change, you were in a comfort zone. You needed information to fully understand what was happening.

Once you understood, you likely recognized that change was happening whether you wanted it or not. At that point, your relationships or productivity may have suffered as you began to question everything, and all sorts of emotions boiled to the surface.

Why me?

Why them?

Why this?

Why now?

What if...?

To weather this stage, you need support that allows you to process through the many emotions that you're feeling. All of those emotions are valid, by the way, and are surfacing to help your subconscious create a new framework that will allow you to move on.

Allow yourself to feel them. Talk with a trusted friend or counselor, or journal about your thoughts and emotions. Don't worry if it doesn't make sense. Just use your journal as a dumping ground for your thoughts.

The processing is important for your growth, so don't try to analyze it; simply allow it. At first, it may feel too scary to allow yourself to feel that deeply. You will live, however, and you'll realize that you are infinitely stronger than you imagined.

Once you've allowed yourself to process your feelings, gradually remind yourself of difficult things you've gone through in the past.

How did you get through those?

Remember strengths you had forgotten. Notice your own small victories on this journey. Force yourself to find something positive in each day, then in each situation. You'll find strengths you didn't know you had.

Eventually, you can decide what you want to keep or discard of the old you and what you want to carry forward as the new you. In this way, you can use every Change Cycle for self-development.

Here's a summary of each stage, along with how to recognize the stages and strategies to help you navigate through them.

Stage One: Resist

In this stage, you experience shock or denial, and you may become immobilized by fear.

Strategies:

- Seek to understand.
- Resist or judge nothing.
- Be unconditionally kind.

Stage Two: Search

In stage two, you're questioning everything as you seek answers, and you may struggle as emotions surface.

Strategies:

- Become an observer of yourself; question, learn, and allow yourself to feel strong emotions.
- Remember tough things you have grown through in the past.
- Schedule fifteen-minute tantrums.
- Find your strengths.
- Problem solve.
- Access trusted support.

Stage Three: Respond

In the final stage, as you fully accept what has occurred, you learn how to adapt. You decide how you'll live your life now, and you begin intentionally creating what's next for you.

Strategies:

- Celebrate your growth, and build on the faith that you've developed in yourself.
- Deliberately choose what you'll leave behind and what you'll carry forward as you create your life from this new perspective.

As you study the cycle and learn strategies to recognize and navigate through change, you'll simplify your life, eliminate struggle, and grow through every change in your life.

Here are some things to keep in mind as you go through change:

- Changing your behavior can feel threatening to others. Share this information with those who are close to you. Let them know you've learned some things that have been helpful to you and may be helpful to them as well. Offer the spirit of learning together to lessen the threat.
- If it feels like someone is sabotaging you, recognize that this feeling is caused by fear, which is part of Stage One. Don't blame them; it's generally a fear that they're not aware of. They may be fearful that if you change, you may leave them, or that your changes would force them, or your relationship with them, to change.
- Just be unconditionally kind with yourself and others during the Change Cycle. Open yourself fully only with a chosen few whom you trust, but share what you want and why you want it with those who are close to you, so they don't become fearful when you begin changing your choices. Understanding will help them move through the cycle, and learning it together can improve your relationship. While they may question your methods or motives in an attempt to avoid change, that doesn't mean they are against you.
- Those who want you to grow will adapt and respond to your changes. Those who don't want the best for you may continue their resistance or even choose to drop out of your life, rather than adapt. That will be their choice. Allow yourself to release them, and you'll gain strength and renewed energy.

Life is change. Growth is optional.

THE NATURAL LAWS

Like all people, you were born with a conscious mind, something possessed by no other species. This unique consciousness is a shared human trait that gives you a singular advantage. You have the power of choice. You can choose how you respond to life — its structure and its content. You can choose a complex life or a simple life.

This ability to choose is far more powerful than most people realize. If you could zoom out and observe how happy, secure people create their lives, you would see that their choices follow a pattern. This pattern is narrowly focused and is practiced consistently. If you studied the pattern, you would see that it also follows known natural laws.

Just as scientists work in concert with proven scientific principles, successful people use the natural laws (which they know they cannot control) and their power of choice (which they know they can control) to create their lives. This powerful combination is available to every one of us; all it takes is understanding and practice. This combination is the key to creating successful outcomes and a satisfying life.

To enhance your life in any area, you can use these natural laws to your advantage. As you build your awareness of them, they will alert you to any practices you are currently doing that are not in harmony with nature. Since these laws all relate to directing energy, you will increase your energy only to the extent that you can align your energy with the natural laws.

If you desire to make a positive change in any area of your life, begin by narrowing your focus and identify a core issue. Then, make a clear choice about that issue.

What is it that you want?

What is it that you never want again?

Figure 3 is a list of the natural laws, along with a brief description of each law and an explanation of how that law relates to you as a person.

Figure 3. Natural Laws

Natural Law	Description	How Law Relates to You
ENERGY	The force behind all life.	You are born with a *life force*, and it is composed of energy.
VIBRATION	All things are composed of atoms, which are in constant motion.	You are made of atoms, and those atoms vibrate at rates that are influenced by your choices.
ATTRACTION	All things gravitate toward like energy.	You attract to you that which matches your vibration.
POLARITY	All things have dual perspectives.	You are free to choose your focus—positive or negative—in each moment.
CREATION	The actions of two things can create a unique third.	Your focus, coupled with your emotions, directs the vibrational energy that, in turn, creates your life.
RHYTHM	All things in nature operate according to a rhythm or cycle.	You will experience cycles of change throughout your lifetime.
CAUSE AND EFFECT	Every action has a reaction.	What appears in your life is the result of your dominant focus and feelings.
RELATIVITY	All things are relative.	All things are relative to your beliefs about them.

Energy

The force behind all life is energy.

You are the physical extension of *nonphysical energy*. This nonphysical energy constitutes an inner part of you that is totally unique and always adores you. This inner you is composed of pure positive energy and is not dependent on your outside circumstances. This inner part, your *spirit*, will guide you toward all things that you truly desire.

Your spirit is the source of your energy. It will give you an accurate reading of your current focus in the form of emotion.

Do you believe that you are meant to feel good?

Do you feel most like yourself when you feel good?

You will understand your source energy by paying attention to how you feel. Your emotions will let you know what you are focused on.

- When you feel good, you have tapped into your energy source and connected with your spirit.
- When you feel bad, you have cut off the source of your energy and disconnected from your spirit.

When you access your spirit, you increase your energy flow.

Vibration

All things are composed of atoms, which are in constant motion.

Thoughts and feelings cause the atoms in your body to vibrate. This vibration projects out into the world like a radio signal.

Your vibrations are the result of what you focus on and how you feel. All that you see, hear, smell, taste, and touch is an interpretation of energy vibrating. That's why two people can respond differently to the same thing.

What you create in your life is the direct result of your vibrational signal. You attract things to you that are a match to your vibration, positive or negative. You have created all that is currently in your life. The dominant thoughts and feelings that you held in the past have set the tone of your vibrational energy, and your signal has attracted like vibrational energy — good and bad. You will attract into your future based on your current signal — always.

Acute stress is usually brief. Stress is enlarged by reliving it or by fearing its return. Those thoughts affect your vibration. Scattered thinking, a cluttered environment, and chaos also lower your vibration. When you clarify your focus, you will raise your vibration, be more resourceful, and remember more.

Have you noticed that when you are clear about what you want most in a situation, you get it?

Decide on the outcome you desire before you enter a situation. Decisions have great vibrational power.

Raising your vibration can be done simply with these three actions:

1. Focus on what you want, not on how you are going to get it.
2. Declutter your environment.
3. Surround yourself with the things that make you feel good.

Attraction

All things gravitate toward like vibration. People, things, and circumstances that match your signal will be drawn to you. Those things that appear in your life are always a match to your dominant vibrations.

Your mind stores information and files it into categories. When you think a thought, your mind searches for a thought to match it—then another, and another. These large sets of matching thoughts are called beliefs. When you have a large set of thoughts, or beliefs, and a new thought matches those thoughts, it expands easily and quickly. That's why it feels more real or why you believe it even if it's not true.

If a new thought does not find supporting thoughts to match it, the new thought feels unreal or unbelievable. That's why changing habits is so difficult. You have a large set of thoughts (beliefs) to support the old habit and haven't yet built a new set of thoughts to support the new habit.

Try these attraction exercises:

- Spend one day noticing only positive aspects.
- Allow yourself to play.
- Hang out with people you find attractive.
- Write down characteristics of your ideal day and your ideal life.
- Spend fifteen minutes every day imagining what you want and appreciate (without the particulars of how it will happen).
- If you find yourself feeling bad, imagine something on your appreciation list, and feel the shift.

Polarity

All things have dual perspectives.

There are two sides to all things: positive and negative.

- There is health and the absence of health
- There is wealth and the lack of wealth
- There is having something and the lack of having it

You have the power to choose, in any moment, which side you will focus on. It's your choice—always.

Since you are free to choose your focus in each moment, focus on what you can control, and then decide what you want to think and feel.

Your responses are caused by your thoughts, not by circumstances or other people.

EVENT + PERCEPTION = RESPONSE

Creation

The actions of two things can create a unique third.

- The joining of male and female contains within it the power to create a third, totally unique, living thing.
- The joining of two chemicals has the power to create a third chemical.
- The joining of your conscious and subconscious minds contains the power to create all that you desire.
- Join your mind with your spirit, and you can access power that is limited only by what you can imagine.

You can deliberately create your life. It begins with clarity.

Follow these eight steps to create what you want.

1. Decide *what* you want to BE, DO, and HAVE in your life.
2. Know *why* you want these things.
3. Write them down.
4. Vividly imagine being, doing, and having your desires.
5. Practice for fifteen minutes, twice a day.
6. Act as if you already have your desires.
7. Look for evidence.
8. Keep the energy flowing.

Whatever holds your dominant attention, coupled with the intensity of the feelings you experience about that, will determine its creation.

FOCUS + FEELINGS = CREATION

Rhythm

All things in nature operate according to a rhythm or cycle.

Life is a series of cycles. We seek ideas and challenges to move us forward. We resist change and hang on to the familiar. We want balance and equilibrium.

Recall the Change Cycle from Step One. Embrace this cycle, for it will be with you throughout your lifetime. When you understand this predictable cycle and have strategies to navigate through it, life will be simpler.

Cause and Effect

Every action has a reaction.

Everything in life responds to the laws. There is no exception. The effects of the laws can be witnessed daily.

Have you noticed that when you feel good, your day goes well?

Have you noticed that when you feel bad, others seem to feel bad?

- Taking action from a good-feeling place results in a positive reaction.
- Taking action from a bad-feeling place results in a negative reaction.

It can be no other way.

Relativity

All things are relative.

Everything is related to something else.

- Your feelings are related to your thoughts.
- Your thoughts are related to your beliefs.
- Your beliefs are related to your habits of thinking.

Your life experience is determined by your relationship with yourself (your energy source, or spirit).

HOW RESULTS ARE CREATED

Your subconscious mind and your conscious mind communicate constantly. Your conscious mind provides information to you via your *thoughts*. Your subconscious mind provides information to you via your *emotions*. Your emotions let you know if what you are focused on is consistent with your energy source.

When you think vivid thoughts and couple them with feelings, positive or negative, your mind stores them as fact, for it cannot tell the difference between real and imagined. Your subconscious must *believe* that the fulfillment of a desire can occur before it will allow it to happen.

Acting-As-If

To create anything new in your life requires building belief. Act *as if* you have your desire, and you will build your set of matching thoughts, your database of belief. With all of your senses, vividly imagine having what you want, and you will attract the means to accomplish it. Your mind will be practicing the new vibration.

- The more you practice, the stronger your vibration will become.
- The stronger your vibration, the stronger your belief.

Frank Lloyd Wright couldn't have said it any clearer:

"The thing always happens that you really believe in. And the belief in a thing makes it happen."

When you vividly imagine, your mind can't tell the difference between real and fantasy. I learned that from studying how successful people reached their goals. I pretended I was a thin person long before the mirror reflected that.

At the time, Jane Fonda was an exercise guru, so I would ask myself: *What would Jane do?*

I envisioned fitting into blue jeans with the back pockets close together.

I couldn't even imagine what that would be like, but I thought:

I'm just going to pretend that I have those blue jeans.

What would really be different?

I'd have the same house, the same pet, the same husband, and the same everything.

Well, maybe I'd walk differently.

I realized that life is lived from the inside out. If you just imagine feeling a certain way and you practice that long enough, eventually, you become that. Acting-as-if is one of the biggest steps to creating lasting change.

I learned that feeling good in my body required regular exercise. Even though I felt like an impostor, I acted like Jane and went to aerobics classes, then step aerobics, kickboxing, Zumba, and all sorts of other exercise classes.

When a friend invited me to a CrossFit workout, I told her that in my wildest dreams, I could not possibly imagine being able to do it. But that dear friend encouraged me and told me that I could, and — lo and behold! — I was able to do it.

Imagine: I had almost stopped myself from embarking on the plan that made me stronger and more fit than anything else I had ever done.

Now, even if I must scale down my workout, I act as if I can do it, and I *do it.*

You'd be amazed at what you are capable of doing.

Act-as-if. Imagine yourself accomplishing your goal, and actually feel what it would be like if you had that goal. Put yourself in the picture by actually visualizing yourself experiencing what you want. Feel it. When you practice feeling it, eventually, your mind begins to buy into it.

Natural Life Principles

Life is not random. Natural phenomena—such as gravity, the changing seasons, and the sunrise and sunset—are all guided by laws that are absolute. They exist whether or not you believe in them.

Humans are also governed by natural principles that can allow us to BE, DO, and HAVE whatever we desire.

In essence: *You get what you think about, and whatever you think about gets bigger.*

The life principles below will be repeated often throughout this book as they lay the foundation for creating your life. Allow yourself time to absorb them, and look for all the ways they show up in your life. Keep an open mind as you test the principles for yourself. Many of the concepts were not taught in traditional schools, so seek additional resources to expand your knowledge. Pay attention to how you feel, and keep a journal to record your insights.

Keep in mind that beliefs are simply repeated thoughts, and habits are repeated behaviors. They are both constructed in the same way.

1. An event occurs, which triggers a thought.
2. Your thought (self-talk) generates a feeling.
3. The thought and feeling generate a response, which leads to an outcome.
4. If the same thought and feeling are repeated over time, a belief is created.
5. Those beliefs, *not the events*, then drive your behavior (response).

You cannot skip or ignore a part of this path; it's how humans work. Review these principles daily, and commit them to memory.

Figure 4 illustrates these life principles and how our thoughts and self-talk lead to events, outcomes, and habits.

Figure 4. Life Principles Sequence of Arrows

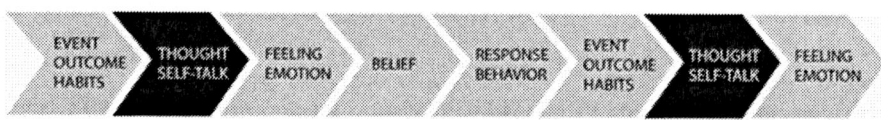

In this sequence, all things are controlled by you except one: EVENTS. Events are those things that are outside your control, such as traffic, weather, or the actions of other people. Notice that your RESPONSE to an event only comes after your THOUGHTS, FEELINGS, and BELIEFS are in place. OUTCOME is listed on the same arrow as EVENT because the sequence doesn't end; it repeats itself over and over.

- Repeating *new thoughts* (positive self-talk) creates *new beliefs*.
- Repeating *new behaviors* (based on your new beliefs) creates *new habits*.

To make any change in how you feel or what you do, begin with your thoughts.

How Thoughts Affect Outcomes

Figure 5 shows the circular effect of how thoughts affect outcomes. You're probably familiar with the vicious cycle of eating and gaining weight.

It goes something like this:

- You tell yourself: *I'm fat.*
- You feel bad.
- You eat something to make yourself feel better.
- You end up gaining weight and telling yourself: *I'm out of control.*
- You feel bad, eat more, and gain more weight.

This is a pattern in our culture that too many people have grown to accept.

But it doesn't have to be that way.

The traditional model of dieting wants you to change your behavior to get results, but we know that doesn't work. If it did, then the very first diet you ever went on would have worked.

Before you can change your behavior, you must address how you feel. To change how you feel, you must change how you think. And to change how you think is as simple as reaching for a good thought.

Figure 5. Thoughts and Outcomes Cycle

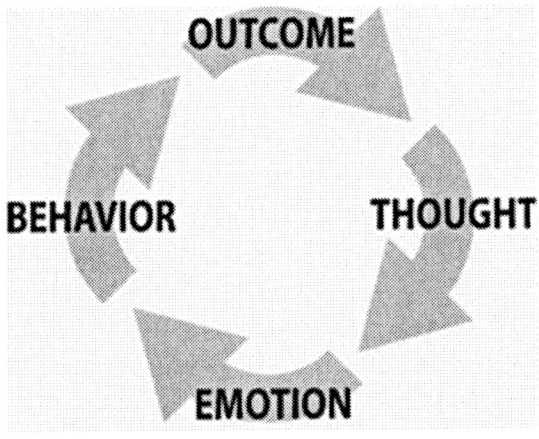

How do you know if you've been thinking good thoughts?

Ask yourself: *How do I feel?*

If you feel good, then you are on the right track. If you feel bad, then reach for a better thought. In the process of reaching for a better thought, you begin to change your outcome.

There's no diet menu or two-week action plan to start on. Change your thoughts, and you will feel better, act differently, and have new outcomes.

If you took the Life Principles Sequence of Arrows (Figure 4, page X) and wound them up like an endless spring coil, you'd get something like this.

Figure 6. Life Principles Spring Coil

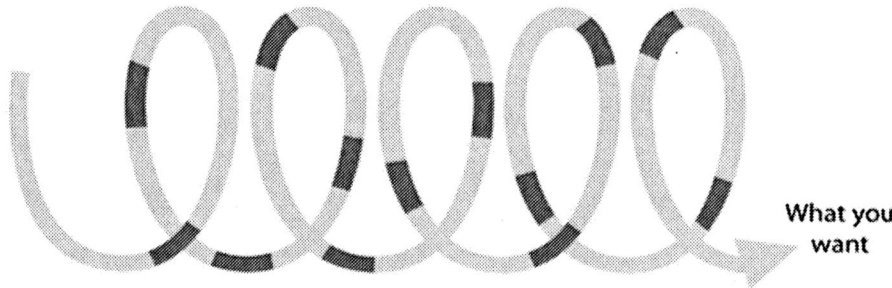

What you want

The dark spots on the spring coil represent self-talk and thoughts. As you move along the coil, every good thought takes you closer to the outcome you desire, and every bad thought slides you back.

Don't worry if you've been feeling down all afternoon; just reach for a better thought. Then, do it again. Keep reaching for better thoughts, one by one, until you feel better. The great thing about this is that you don't have to wait to get better outcomes because they always happen after each better thought.

What is that better outcome?

You feel better, and you begin attracting more positive experiences into your life.

Just reach for thoughts you *can* reach, even if they're not extremely happy thoughts. The key is simply to find thoughts that you can believe in that moment, and that focus you on something more positive than any negative thought you had been thinking.

What you want is always going to change based on your perspective at the time. Once you get one thing that you wanted, you'll want something else, and that's okay. Your patience with this process will pay off because you won't be backtracking on this journey ever again.

"We are what we repeatedly do. Excellence, then, is not an act but a habit."

Aristotle said this over 2,300 years ago, and it couldn't be more true today. Those who excel in life don't just excel in one area; they excel in many areas of their lives because being excellent is not a one-time thing; it's an everyday occurrence.

And what makes them excel?

It's the way they think and what they think.

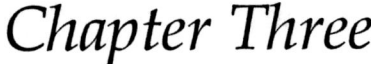

Chapter Three

A Fresh Start

During the two years that I remained separated from my husband, I was very angry that our relationship hadn't worked out. I felt like I had put my whole life on hold for him and, consequently, had not developed my own career. Instead, here I was doing medical transcription. Feeling that anger fueled my resolve to exercise, which, in turn, gave me energy. I began to feel better about myself once again. The exercise also helped me to stay off drugs and to get reacquainted with myself.

Shortly after that, I met someone new. Ron (who is now my husband) had been a musician for twenty-five years prior to returning to college. He was unlike anyone I'd ever met, and I felt good every time I was around him. When I met him, he was playing in a band, he had nothing but a fifty-dollar car and a new college degree, and he was going to move from Colorado to Florida to start his career.

In spite of the fact that a lot of my friends thought I was completely nuts, I moved with Ron to Florida, sight unseen. I adored him, and it just felt right.

Even though I had never imagined that I would live anywhere other than Colorado, had never lived any place east of the Mississippi, and had no concept of what that might be like, I remember being surprised that my friends seemed shocked at my decision to leave everything I'd known and loved for so long.

"Linda, what are you doing? Are you crazy, running away with a bass player?"

I was rather cavalier about the whole thing.

"What's the big deal? Florida is in the United States. How different could it be?"

I was ready for adventure and a fresh start in my life.

As it turned out, moving from Boulder, Colorado, to Melbourne Beach, Florida, was like relocating to another planet. I was absolutely miserable and completely unprepared for the huge adjustments I would need to make. All at once, I found myself with no family, no friends, and nothing familiar.

Everything in Florida felt so foreign: The landscape was completely flat; the air was so thick that I could touch it; the humidity was so heavy that it made me slump from the weight; I couldn't breathe; I couldn't tell north from south because there was nothing visible for me to set my sights on; and I couldn't tell what season it was because they all seemed the same.

I missed the snow, I missed the leaves changing colors, and I desperately missed my mountains, my friends, and my family. I hated Florida, and I feared falling into the depression that I had vowed never again to experience.

But even though, in some ways, I felt very, very bad, I had reasons to stay. I was finally with the right man, and I felt loved, unconditionally. I had to find a way to make it work.

I tried using my acting-as-if tools, but I needed much more. I used to joke that I had a low tolerance for feeling bad. While that was true, I now understood that the tools I had relied on were not creating happiness for me there. Though I hated to admit it, I realized that I was the common denominator in my depressive episodes and that perhaps Florida was not to blame.

Since I wanted a fresh life and there was a college there, I decided to go to graduate school. I was going to find a career for myself and create a life that I loved.

One thing I realized about my marriage with my ex-husband was that I really wanted what he had. I wanted to love my work and have the world pay me well for it. I had gotten jealous of him, actually. I didn't want to be second-in-command anymore.

For the first time in my life, I actually became assertive.

I decided: *I'm going to get a master's degree. That's going to be my ticket to a real career.*

I needed my own work.

As I look back, I wonder: *If I had been more confident about my body earlier in my life, would I have had more confidence in my abilities?*

I think I would have.

My degree program in grad school was very challenging, and I put a lot of effort into installing exercise into my routine to relieve stress and build my confidence (a practice that has continued for many, many years). I finally felt like my body wasn't constantly on the verge of being out of control.

When I got my degree, I was thrilled. For the first time in my life, I knew exactly what job I wanted. When an employee assistance program (EAP) counselor position suddenly appeared as an open posting and I didn't meet the qualifications because I wasn't a licensed mental health counselor, I didn't let that stop me. I wanted it so badly that I talked my way into it, and they gave it to me.

At the same time, after two years of having my head in a book, I looked up and realized: *I'm still in Florida, and I still don't like it.*

So I sought out counseling to get some help.

When I found a therapist and began to learn how my thinking had been trapping me, I initially scoffed at the idea.

How could this be my fault?

To prove her wrong, I decided to test what she was telling me. I began tracking my thoughts and feelings, and I discovered that my thinking did contain errors. I made assumptions, I generalized, I judged, and I blamed.

So many things that I had thought I never did, I was doing daily.

"But I'm a good person," I told my therapist.

"That's exactly why it feels so bad. Those thoughts make you feel bad because that's not who you really are."

Now, I'm eternally grateful to that psychologist. She helped me to see how to change my thinking and that my happiness had nothing to do with where I lived. Even though, at times, I was resentful and still wanted to blame Florida, as I practiced choosing new thoughts, I felt better. And that's when things really started happening for me.

I realized that I hadn't really accepted my divorce and gone through a grieving process. The therapist helped me to learn about the Change Cycle and taught me the importance of processing all of the emotions that I had stuffed down inside of myself for so long. That's when I learned that you don't get to skip any stage. It was a difficult process, but she gave me tools, and I used them.

Step Three:
Practice Feeling Good

Even if all you do is focus on what you want instead of what you don't want, you'll get rid of a whole bunch of extraneous thoughts.

FEELINGS AND FOCUS

Most people are pretty clear about what they *don't want* but are very unclear about what they *do want.* (I felt that way too.) As you begin to understand how your mind works, you'll discover that focusing on what you don't want actually creates more of it.

Have you ever been on a diet and gained weight?

It's very common, and it happened to me. Every time I went on one of those diets, the less I lost and the more I gained.

Why?

It's an equation; you get what you focus on.

When you're on a diet, do you think about food or weight more often than you did before?

If your answer is yes, you're setting yourself up to gain more (or want more). That's a pretty important thing to know.

If you diet often, I'll bet you mostly think about weight or food. That's the fatal flaw of the dieting approach. We end up being focused on the very thing that we do not want, and that attaches us to the problem.

Another challenge about changing your body is that you're going to encounter life along the way. For a lot of people, the biggest challenge they have is keeping their focus on what they want. From celebrations at work to social situations to family expectations, it seems like there's always something to derail us.

Here's an example of focusing on what you want:

I want to be thin.

Why?

Because being thin will mean that I'm healthier.

Why do you want to be healthier?

So I'll have more energy.

Why do you want more energy?

So I can take care of my children better, do better at work, and not feel tired all the time, and I can have some fun.

Clarify what you want, and be as specific as you can be. This will help you create a compelling image to focus upon and feel good about. That way, you'll enjoy focusing on what you want, and those thoughts will grow and help you to achieve it.

As you progress, the clarity of knowing what you want will also alert you when you are getting off track, so it's important to pay attention to how you feel. As you focus on the things you want, you may also notice a shift in how you define them.

Let your energy guide you, and just be as honest and specific as you can be. That may take some practice if you've focused on what you don't want for a long time. Just remember that when you focus on what you don't want, it attracts like energy and gets bigger. You then prevent yourself from getting what you truly want.

Define what you want, and focus your thoughts and intentions on those things. ***If you feel bad, it's your emotions alerting you that you're focused on what you don't want.*** Practice focusing on what you want, and refine your choices as you progress.

Figure 7. What You Focus on Gets Bigger

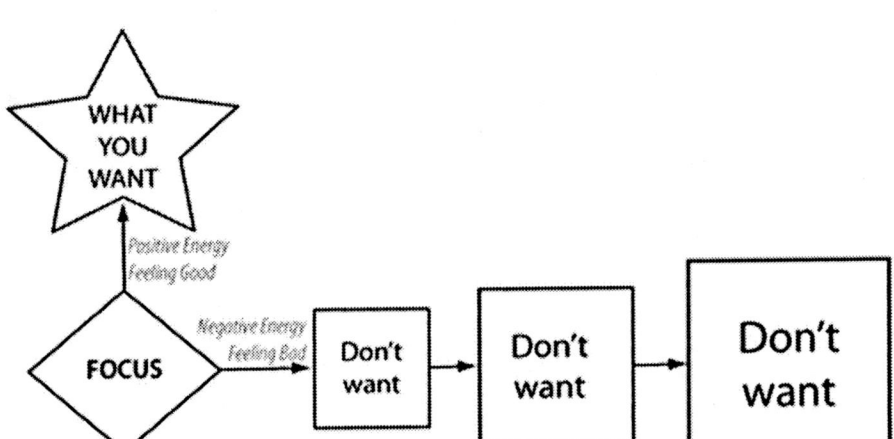

When you feel good, you are focused on what you want.

Do you remember a time when you felt good?

What were you doing?

Maybe you were having dinner with friends. Maybe you were on vacation. Maybe it has been a long time since you've felt good. But you have felt good before. It may have been a temporary feeling as you sat down to watch a movie with a fresh bowl of popcorn and a cold soda, but you felt good.

Can you remember the last time you felt bad?

(Was it when the movie ended and you realized that you had just eaten four cups of buttered popcorn and drunk forty-eight ounces of soda?)

You have the skills to know when something feels good and when it doesn't. When you feel bad, you need to change your focus to what you want. To make sure that your focus stays where you want it, remember to set a clear intention.

Set the intention to have what you want.

I want to be healthy.

I have the intention, right now, to be healthy.

The intention will guide your choices. Your feelings will guide your focus.

ENERGY FLOW AND THOUGHTS

Do you believe you are meant to feel good?

Do you feel most like yourself when you feel good?

When you feel joy, you are feeling your spirit, your life force. Think of it as an inner you. It is composed of pure positive energy and is not dependent on your outside circumstances. When you access your spirit, you increase your energy flow. **When you feel joy, you have tapped into your energy source.** When you have bad feelings—like anger, guilt, or shame—you have cut off the source of your energy.

Have you noticed that when you add doubt or cynicism to a good thought, your energy drops?

I'm doing well now, but what if it doesn't last?

I'm better, but I still have so far to go.

We do it to ourselves, simply by shifting our focus to what we don't want. And every time we shift to what we don't want, we halt our forward progress and cut off the flow from our spirit, which is our energy source.

This is quite normal. You have patterns of thinking that you have developed over time. You may not currently realize what you habitually focus upon. That's why practice is essential in this area.

Familiarize yourself with your levels of energy.

When are they:

- High?
- Low?
- Flat?

Notice how you feel when you focus upon certain objects or topics. Notice whether you focus on what you want or on what you don't want. Begin the practice of identifying what you want most in each life situation, and focus on what you want without being attached to how you will get it.

All things in life either support or deplete you. Eliminate those things that deplete you, and allow yourself to be filled with what supports you. Let your practice be to keep perfecting your ability to feel good.

In order to feel good, it is critical to be aware of what you think and to notice the messages that you tell yourself.

The voice in your head that reminds you to pick up the dry cleaning

The voice that tells you keep going

The voice that tells you to slow down

What is that voice?

It is merely what you decide it is. It is what you decide to think. There are thinking habits that can block your energy (negative habits of thinking) and those that can create energy (positive habits of thinking).

Eliminating Energy Drains

What you take in with your eyes, ears, nose, mouth, and touch affects you. Those things that do not support you drain your energy.

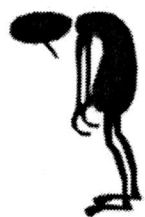

Some examples of energy drains are:

- Unmet needs
- Negative thoughts
- Trying to control things you can't control
- Clutter
- Lack of systems to deal with things like change, conflict, and chaos

What are the things that you complain about yet have done nothing to correct?

Those things are costing you:

- Peace of mind
- Patience
- Time
- Money
- Space

Use the following list to help you identify your energy drains. Write down all the things that you currently tolerate in each of these areas:

- Home
- Work
- Money
- Friends
- Relatives
- Car
- Education
- Recreation
- Errands
- Me
- Pets
- Yard

Creating Space

There's a theory that if you own things you don't value, then those things don't value you either. Energetically, you will be creating a negative energy match. That's why it's important to rid your environment of things you no longer value. If you feel guilty, just remember that there are plenty of people who have very little and would be thrilled to have the opportunity to value what you consider worthless.

All that you have acquired in your life is made up of energy, and it all takes up space in your life. If you have things that you no longer value, consider that *dead space*; it's taking up room in your life and adding nothing.

Not only that, but *if your life is too full, you're actually preventing new things from coming to you.* There simply isn't any room for them.

If you find yourself saying that you have no time, consider this:

Having no time is an indicator that you are too full to make a significant shift.

Essentially, you are living in an *expired paradigm*; you have expanded as much as you can within that particular framework in your life. Just as very little change can occur in a crowded space, when you have learned all you can about something, you are essentially full and cannot add more.

You become stuck.

When you eliminate the meaningless clutter in your life, you allow much larger shifts to occur because there is sufficient space for movement. In fact, change rushes in to fill the void. So, when you remove clutter *and* you're clear about your vision, things often begin happening quickly.

When you're clear about why you're here, life is simply about choosing your focus and keeping stuff out of your way. When you have things in your life that no longer serve you, or things that actually annoy you, your frustration will squander precious energy for no purpose. These are your energy drains. Plug those energy drains, and you release positive energy that can be utilized to move you toward your vision.

CLUTTER = DECREASED ENERGY

CREATING SPACE = INCREASED ENERGY

Thoughts That Drain Energy (Messages That Cause You to Feel Like a Victim)

Here are some common habits of thinking that can drain your energy:

ABSOLUTE THINKING: You see things as black or white. If your performance falls short of perfect, you see yourself as a failure.

If I don't follow my diet exactly, I might as well just forget it and eat the whole cake.

I had one extra cookie, so I might as well eat the whole bag.

GENERALIZING: You see a single negative event as a never-ending pattern of defeat. (Hint: You often use words like *always* or *never*.)

I never get what I want. (Really? Never?)

When you repeat those thoughts long enough, your mind eventually believes them as if they're facts. They're not facts, of course, but that's how your mind records them. Remember, repetition creates belief.

FILTERING: You pick out a negative detail and dwell on it. You begin to see the world through a lens that has been darkened by that detail, like the drop of ink that discolors the entire beaker of water.

DISQUALIFYING POSITIVES: You reject positive experiences by insisting that they don't count. This allows you to justify your negative belief even when it's contradicted by a positive experience.

ASSUMING: You arbitrarily make a conclusion even though there is no evidence to support it.

MIND-READING: You think that you know what someone else is thinking, and you base your response on that assumption.

I know what's going on in your brain, so I'm going to base my actions on that.

If you're human, you've probably done this. (The embarrassing truth is that I've made big life decisions based on mind-reading.)

Consider this: Do you mind-read positively or negatively?

Most people mind-read negatively. (They imagine the worst thoughts in the mind of the other person.) This, of course, just makes them feel bad and does nothing to the other person.

Since you're making it up anyway, why not make up something that feels good?

You could think: *Gee, that person over there thinks I'm pretty terrific.*

Repeatedly imagining negative thoughts about another person eventually develops a negative belief, which then feels like a fact. We typically don't check it out; we simply act upon our belief as if it's a fact.

ANTICIPATING DOOM: You anticipate that things will turn out badly, and you feel convinced that your prediction is an already-established fact.

I know what's going to happen in the future; therefore, I'm going to base my actions on that.

That's like feeling bad on the way to the dentist.

I'm going to feel bad now, just in case.

It doesn't make any logical sense, yet we do it all the time. The truth is that we could imagine things turning out well, but we often don't do that. We catastrophize.

Why?

To protect ourselves.

What we don't realize is that it can become a bad habit.

EXAGGERATING: You magnify the importance of things, or you inappropriately shrink things until they seem tiny. (We often exaggerate our goof-ups and shrink our good qualities.)

EMOTIONALIZING: You assume that your feelings reflect the way things are.

I feel it, so it must be true.

I feel it; therefore, it's a fact.

This is actually backwards. ***You feel it because you thought it. If you can change the thought, you can change how it feels.*** (Of course, if you've practiced a negative thought for so long that it has become a belief, then this won't happen immediately.)

EXPECTATIONS: You try to motivate yourself with shoulds and shouldn'ts. You set yourself up with expectations that other people should or should not behave in certain ways. The results of these demands are guilt, shame, resentment, rebelliousness, anger, disappointment, or depression.

LABELING: Instead of telling yourself: *I made a mistake*, you tell yourself: *I'm a fool*. When applied to other people who irritate you, you tell yourself: *He's a jerk*. When I was growing up and I labeled myself as clumsy and fat, I became more of that. Eliminating negative labels opens the door to revise how you see yourself and others.

TAKING THINGS PERSONALLY: You see yourself as the cause of some event for which you were not responsible or over which you did not have control.

If only I had paid more attention to my brother, he would not have had the car wreck.

These are called victim messages, and we've probably all used at least some of these. They keep us stuck because they reinforce beliefs over which we have no control.

Poor me!

This is a sure way to keep yourself in a negative cycle.

Thoughts That Create Energy (Messages That Empower You)

THE ONLY PERSON WHO HAS TO LIKE ME IS ME. I don't necessarily like everyone I know, so why should I expect everyone to like me?

MY MISTAKES ARE MY GREATEST TEACHERS. The only people who never make mistakes are those who never try. I will accept mistakes in myself and the mistakes that others make.

I ACCEPT MYSELF AND OTHERS UNCONDITIONALLY. Just like me, the people who do things I don't like are trying to cope, and they use whatever skills they have.

I ACHIEVE PEACE BY GIVING UP MY NEED FOR CONTROL. I will survive if things are different from how I want them to be. I can accept myself the way I am.

I ASSUME TOTAL RESPONSIBILITY FOR MY LIFE. I am responsible for how I feel and what I do. It is not the responsibility of other people to change so that I can feel better.

I AM MORE POWERFUL THAN OUTSIDE EVENTS. Things usually go just fine, and when they don't, I can handle it. I don't have to waste my energy worrying.

EVEN IN THE FACE OF CHALLENGE, I ALWAYS TRY. Avoiding a task does not give me any opportunities for success or joy, but trying does. I might not be able to do everything, but I can do something.

I RELY ONLY ON MYSELF FOR DECISIONS, CHOICES, AND SELF-CARE. I don't need someone else to take care of my problems. I am capable of making my own decisions.

MY PAST DOES NOT DETERMINE MY FUTURE. I don't have to be a certain way because of what has happened in the past. Every day is a new day.

JUST BECAUSE I'M NOT CONCERNED DOESN'T MEAN I DON'T CARE. I can't solve other people's problems for them. They are capable and can solve their own problems.

I CAN BE FLEXIBLE AND ANTICIPATE THE BEST. There is no one-and-only best way. I trust that things will turn out well.

You could also use shorter versions, such as:

- Everybody doesn't have to like me.
- It's okay to make a mistake.
- Other people are okay, and I'm okay.
- I don't have to control things.
- I am responsible for my day.
- I can handle it when things go wrong.
- I can be flexible.
- I can change.
- I am capable.

Shifting to a Better Thought

You are most resourceful when you feel good.

Things that are now effortless for you, like driving a car, required attention and repetition while you were learning them. Feeling good is no different.

What happens physically and emotionally when you think about the things that make you feel good?

Remember the section about focusing on what you want?

When you were on a traditional diet, how did you feel?

Did you feel satisfied and content, or did you feel deprived?

What was your focus?

Was it on *food* and what you could and could not eat?

Or were you focused on how much *exercise* you had to do?

We all know the basic equation:

CALORIES IN - CALORIES OUT = WEIGHT LOSS

Perhaps you were focused on your calorie intake.

But how did you *feel*?

If you felt good, you probably kept it up and lost some weight.

When you had a bad day and felt bad, what happened to your diet?

This is where the slip-ups happen.

When things change, you must have a good way of coping with those changes. Practice reaching for a better thought. You can't be expected to go from angry to enthusiastic by thinking a happy thought, but you can go from angry to mildly frustrated or even neutral by examining your thoughts.

When you are feeling sad, angry, jealous, or worried, look at the thoughts that are draining your energy. Remember the Change Cycle, recognize where you are, and know that you're going to be okay.

Don't go looking for the thought that caused what you don't want. That would be a bit like taking a turn down a dead-end road. Most of us drive down to the end of the road just to make sure the sign was telling the truth. Then, we get really stuck. As soon as you see the sign, turn the car around. Identify what you want or where you're going again. That will help pull your emotions back up to feeling better.

Just turn the car around by finding a thought that feels better.

Positive thoughts don't have to be "yippee!" happy thoughts. Just reach for a thought that you can reach.

When I was feeling at my darkest, I learned how to do this, and the thought I reached for was:

I'm still breathing.

That's not a very high thought.

My next one was:

I'm not bleeding.

I wasn't reaching very far.

My cat loves me.

Those were my three reliable positive thoughts.

You can reach a little higher. Please do. Just reach for a thought that's close by, and it will pull you away from the cliff of negativity so you can refocus.

The good news is that your mind is linear and can focus on only one thing at a time. When you shift from a bad thought to a better thought, you'll feel better. It may take some practice to get to that better feeling place, but you can get there, one thought at a time.

Figure 8 shows how a different thought can lead to a different outcome. Just like the Life Principles Spring Coil (Figure 6, page X), every good thought will take you closer to where you want to be.

Figure 8. Reaching for a New Outcome

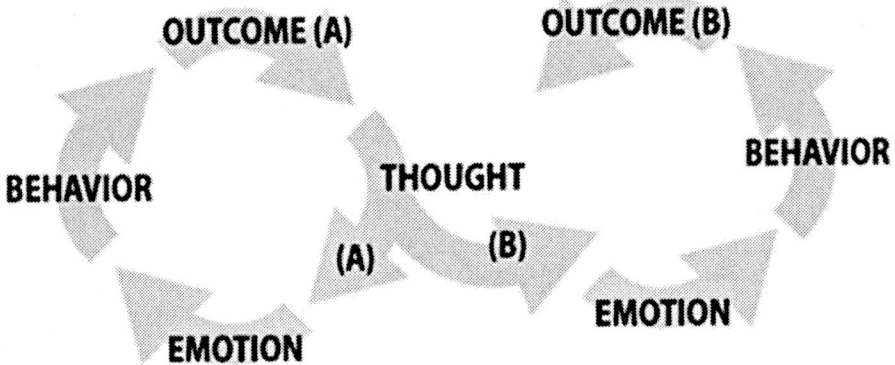

BELIEFS AND BEHAVIOR

It's very common to hang onto the past. We beat ourselves up, place blame, feel loss. We generalize our experiences and label ourselves as a result.

Forgiving Yourself and Moving Forward

To *Leave That Behind* is to look only forward and not relive past mistakes. The truth is, it's not your fault.

How do you forgive yourself?

I recommend these steps:

1. Identify Your Story

This is the story you tell yourself about why you can't have what you really want.

2. Challenge Your Rules

This is the list of things by which you judge yourself.

3. Label Your Dreams

Be honest.

What's the BIG thing you really want?

(Hint: It may not be a *thing*.)

4. Start an *Appreciation Journal*

(Oprah called it a gratitude journal.)

Each day, record three to five things that you appreciate. Because you have to look for them, this trains your mind to find things to appreciate.

Just find some little things that you appreciate in your life.

How does that feel?

It should feel good.

This is a tiny example of how you can help yourself to feel good, any time you want, with just a thought. It has nothing to do with outside circumstances. You can do it on your own.

5. Replace Victim Messages With Power Messages

I can handle this.

I can be flexible.

I can change.

These things are all within my own control.

6. Partner With Your Subconscious

Your subconscious is a whole lot bigger than your conscious mind, so don't ignore it.

There is a theory that says, "Feel the fear, and do it anyway."

I think that's a really hard way to do things.

Instead, tell your subconscious:

I know that you want to protect me, but here's the deal: I really am going to have what I want. I promise you, I won't do anything risky. No more 'lose twenty pounds in a month' schemes.

Just have a little conversation with it.

Your subconscious exists to protect you, so if you've become disappointed with diets before, then it's going to say:

Oh, no, no, no. Who do you think you are?

That's just because it doesn't want you to go through that disappointment again. The good news is that you don't have to get rid of any of the database that your subconscious has built up. Just honor it.

Thank you for recording all of that for me. Here's where I'm going. I am going to have this thing. Partner with me, and I promise you that I'll keep you informed and I'll keep myself safe.

Your Personal Belief System

We all have a personal belief system. It began when we were very young and was fed by those who cared for us. As we grew up, we began to add information from other sources and perhaps modified our original beliefs. These beliefs form an internal roadmap that your life experience will follow exactly, unless you consciously choose to alter the map.

The beliefs you hold about yourself are pivotal in determining how much of your potential you will achieve. You will not move beyond these beliefs. Just as a map is only useful if it includes the locations to which we want to travel, your internal roadmap will only let you travel to those destinations it has recorded as accessible.

Limiting beliefs define the boundaries of your internal roadmap. Your subconscious will send danger signals in an attempt to stop you from moving beyond your perceived limits, whether they are about yourself or the world.

Examples of limiting beliefs:

- Nothing is easy.
- I'm not as smart, so I have to work twice as hard.
- I always struggle with my weight.

Emotions become attached to beliefs and can add to their intensity, making it difficult to identify the thought.

Examples of attached emotions:

- Fear
- Anger
- Frustration
- Helplessness
- Worry
- Jealousy
- Envy
- Hopelessness

Language you habitually use is an indicator of your beliefs.

How do you talk about your situation or life in general?

Examples of language that can indicate limiting beliefs:

- I'm no good at change.
- I just don't have any willpower.
- I'll never be…(healthy, fit, rich, happy, married).

Behaviors are indicators of your beliefs.

Limiting beliefs cause limiting behaviors, like:

- Being fearful of changes in schedule or circumstance
- Overuse of food, alcohol, or shopping
- Performing below your capability

Of course, your behavior naturally follows your thoughts, feelings, and language and further cements the limiting belief in your life. Your behavior may seem quite logical to you because it is supported by the first three elements. *But your behavior is simply the limiting belief in action, creating things that match it.*

How to Move Past Your Limiting Beliefs

To understand your belief system, look at your life. It will be an exact reflection.

You could try to uncover and eliminate all your limiting beliefs, language, feelings, and behaviors, but it would be difficult, if not impossible, to find them all.

There is a better way to shift your beliefs. Remember, your mind is linear; that is, it can only think one thought at a time. When you place your full attention on one thought, in that moment, your mind is aware of nothing else.

How do you change a belief?

There is a theory that you have to get rid of beliefs, but that's not really true. You have to refocus your mind. If you have a negative thought, and you install a positive thought that you repeatedly focus on instead, the negative thought will eventually fade away due to the lack of attention. Recognize your belief, and you can change it. Just focus on your new thought long enough for it to become a belief.

If you try to get rid of a negative belief, you'll focus on the negative thought, so it's going to get bigger, not smaller. That's the fallacy with getting rid of a belief. It will functionally keep you attached to it. So don't even worry about getting rid of beliefs, simply install different thoughts. It's much easier.

Steps to changing a belief:

1. Stop acting or thinking on the basis of the old belief.
2. Substitute a new (more rational and personally meaningful) belief for the old one.
3. Act in light of the new belief.
4. Continue to behave in the rational new way, *even if it feels phony* to act this new way. This will cause the new belief to become real and a part of your natural behavior (as long as you keep practicing). That's how new positive habits are created.

The Focus Wheel

Figure 9 illustrates how one thought can build upon another in order to expand your beliefs and thus allow you to achieve the outcome you desire.

Figure 9. The Focus Wheel

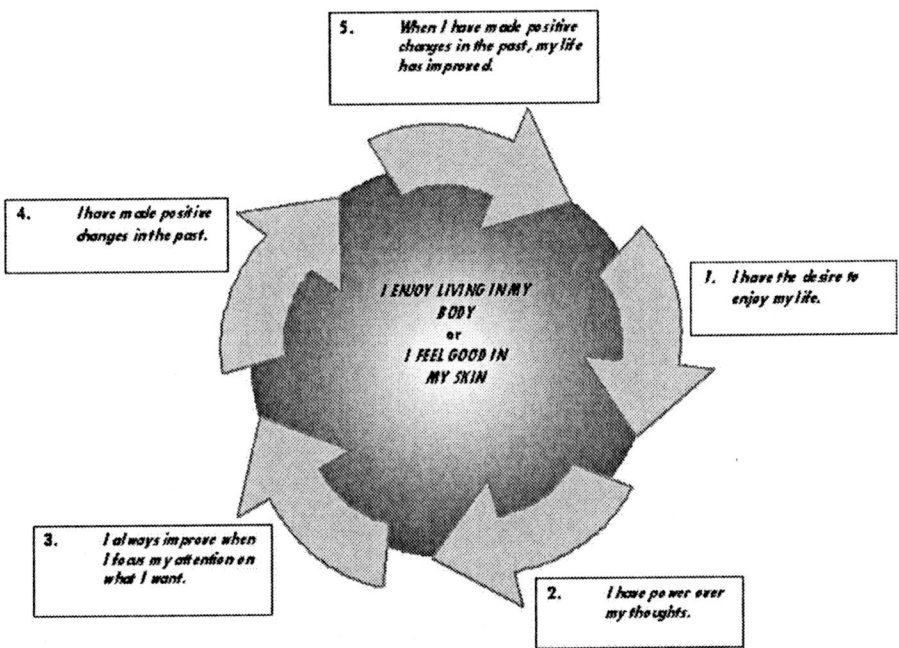

Repeated behaviors become habits. Repeated thoughts become beliefs. With practice, you can develop new habits and new beliefs.

To create your own focus wheel:

1. Write the outcome you desire in the center of the circle.
2. Begin in the first box with general statements that you believe.

3. Work your way clockwise around the circle with related beliefs.
4. Make your statements more specific as you progress around the circle.

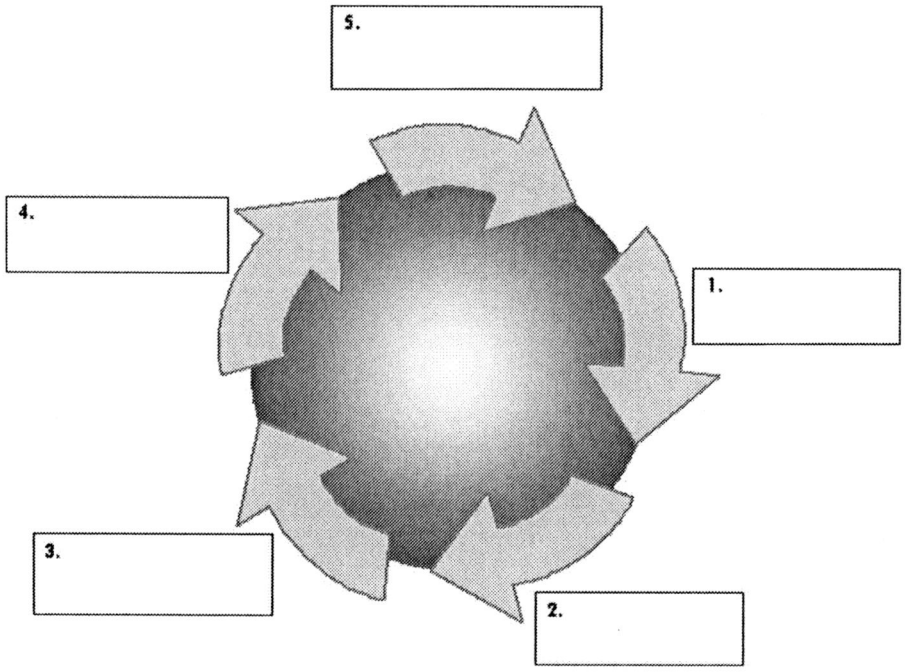

Using Self-Talk to Change Old Habits

"Change your Habits."

It sounds clichéd.

We've all heard it before. It's the basis for the traditional weight-loss diet.

As you saw in the previous diagrams, outcomes and habits are the result of our responses and behaviors, which are the result of what we tell ourselves. Remember, trying to change a behavior with willpower doesn't work. But change your self-talk, and your habits will change.

If you have negative self-talk, you'll have negative feelings, which will build negative beliefs that will cause a negative outcome. It's an equation. It can't be any other way.

Most diets would have you start with the behavior. Change the behavior, and then everything else will follow. Aside from the fact that this doesn't work, I think it's a whole lot easier to start with self-talk. It doesn't require special shoes. You don't have to sweat. But you do have to be aware of your thought patterns.

The messages that you tell yourself all day ultimately drive your behavior, right?

Your mind is actually in charge.

Sometimes it feels like your inner robot (what you do habitually or automatically, without thinking) is running the show, but you actually use your mind to make those decisions. You just don't notice because it's habitual.

If you understand what your thought patterns are, you can reprogram them. (When I learned this, I realized that I had some thought patterns that were keeping me stuck in unhealthy cycles.)

Figure 10 shows how positive self-talk can help you create and sustain healthy habits and negative self-talk creates or sustains unhealthy habits.

Figure 10. Changing Your Self-Talk

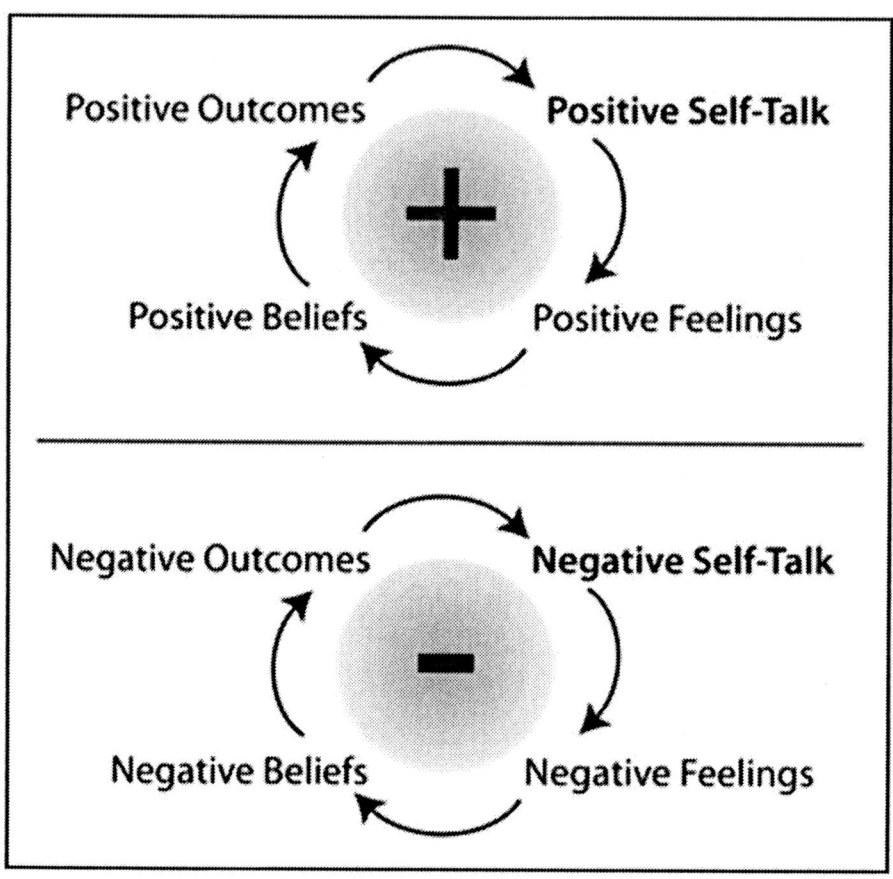

Don't be too hard on yourself regarding change. Instead, try to become an observer of yourself.

Ask yourself:

What habits do I need to change?

Do I see them in many areas of my life?

Can I find any humor there?

As an observer of yourself, you can see how and why your habits and responses are formed. You'll notice that your responses are caused by your thoughts, not by events, and that all of your habits began with a positive intent.

As you repeat new behaviors, you'll create new habits.

As you repeat thoughts you'll create new beliefs.

NEW BEHAVIORS + NEW BELIEFS = PERMANENT CHANGE

The Behavior Bop

When you were a child, did you ever hit a bop bag?

When you punch the top of the bag, it responds by moving in the direction you punched. Because it's weighted, the base of the bag does not move and determines where the bag will stay. Even though the top of the bag moves, it pops back into place, right where you started.

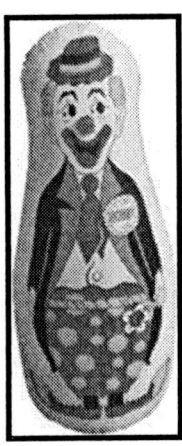

Imagine that your behavior is the top of the bag, and your thinking is the base. Trying to change your behavior without changing how you think is like punching the top of the bag and expecting it to come back up in a different place.

If you want to permanently change the location of the top of the bop bag (your behavior), you must move the base of the bag (your thinking). Otherwise, you create only temporary change.

Changing any habit that doesn't serve you can be done in the same way. Unhealthy eating isn't the only habit that you may want to change. A healthy lifestyle means a healthy body, mind, and spirit. Reviewing your energy drains will give you a place from which to shift your focus.

Practice Being Healthy

Creating a healthy life takes practice, and practice can be implemented immediately. Just as the word *practice* implies, you must do something repeatedly in order to learn or acquire proficiency. As you practice being healthy, you will become better at replacing unhealthy habits with healthy ones.

How do you do that?

By focusing on what you want, choosing positive thoughts, and paying attention to how you feel.

The process works in every situation and every circumstance.

You may need to reinforce your intentions, especially at first. You can strengthen your resolve by recommitting daily.

Affirmations—written on index cards and placed where you'll see them often—can help to keep your intention in your awareness and imprint its importance on your subconscious mind.

Here are few examples:

- *I create my life moment by moment.*
- *I willingly offer the world my best.*

- *My past does not determine my future.*
- *I forgive myself for not seeing clearly.*
- *I am free to be the me that I love.*
- *I believe in myself.*
- *I love myself no matter what.*
- *All is well.*
- *I'm grateful for the future that I'm creating.*

Let your dominant focus be on *feeling good*. **You have far more to offer the world by feeling good than by feeling bad.**

Dealing with Fear and Anger

Remember: We live in a culture that will tempt you to demand quick results. When you feel restless and impatient, recognize that those feelings are created by thoughts that are likely to awaken fear.

What do you do when you're afraid?

- If you tend to flee, then you'll want to give up and seek another route to happiness.
- If you tend to fight, then you'll want to get angry and force a quick solution.

Either response will shut off access to the source of your energy and halt your forward progress.

There is a better way. Instead of awakening fear, install the regular practice of taking the smallest step you can think of to move forward.

Do you feel like quitting?

Call a supportive friend, read something inspirational, or research one more website.

Do you feel like getting angry at your boss?

Take a brisk walk, or drink a large glass of water.

In other words, there is always something within your control that will put you back in charge of your life.

This journey is about developing belief in yourself. Taking small actions, thinking small thoughts, and noticing small moments will keep you in charge of your life, which is the critical component of self-esteem and a healthy lifestyle. Remember that it is an equation, not a chance happening. You can do this.

Continuously seek to find the best-feeling place, and you will forever evolve through change.

Remember: Change happens moment by moment.

- Your mind builds beliefs based on repeated thoughts.
- Your mind can't distinguish between reality and fantasy.
- Vivid imagining builds belief.
- Acting-as-if builds belief.
- For permanent change, beliefs must support behavior.

Narrow Your Focus, and Do the Smallest Thing

Every day, we're bombarded by so much input that our minds can be overflowing with thoughts.

A fascinating study showed that high-performance athletes actually think about half as many thoughts as the rest of us do. They have trained their minds to focus so narrowly on what they want that they have eliminated all extraneous thoughts.

I think that's astounding.

That's what allows them to achieve the amazing things that they do.

You can train yourself to do that too.

Can you do it as well as an athlete?

I don't know, but you can certainly try.

Even if all you do is focus on what you want instead of what you don't want, you'll get rid of a whole bunch of extraneous thoughts.

Chapter Four

The Sticking Point

Learning how to change my thinking had led me to a whole new realm of deliberately creating my life, and I was very proud of myself. I now had a master's degree and a profession that I loved. After years of working hard but never feeling successful, I finally felt like I had control over my own success.

My focus was no longer on managing my weight; it was now on feeling good. I had begun to work with clients by that time, and it was very important to me to be my best for them.

My new profession motivated me to keep learning and growing. For the first time in my adult life, I felt like a peer with other professionals. In my career as an EAP counselor, I finally felt like I was doing work that mattered.

I also experienced the exhilaration of wanting to excel at something. Being new to this field and having peers who were experienced mental health counselors, I was committed to doing whatever it took to be good at assessing, making the right referrals, and (especially) short-term counseling.

I soon learned that to do that effectively required very targeted tools, so I became a practitioner of neurolinguistic programming (NLP) and studied short-term therapy techniques. The tools worked, and I was thrilled! For the first time in my life, I was being praised for work that was meaningful to me. I experienced a level of self-esteem that I had never known.

At that point, my reasons for eating well and exercising shifted. Throughout my adjustment to being in Florida, I had kept up my regimen mostly out of a fear of becoming depressed. Now, however, my eating and exercise habits seemed to make a difference in my ability to be a good counselor. If I didn't exercise or if I ate fatty foods, I felt sluggish and dull, and I wasn't much good to my clients. When I exercised and ate light, I felt sharp and resourceful. That was a huge shift for me because, previously, I'd only been aware of how my weight affected me.

As long as I focused on my newfound career, I felt terrific. I could ignore where I lived and bask in the glory of being praised for my work. I began to lead seminars and discovered that I enjoyed public speaking and training small groups.

There was, however, one little sticking point that remained: Even though I had constructed a whole new life and career in spite of my location, I still carried blame toward this place where I lived, and this place where I lived was full of people.

But that's no problem because I always see people as people...right?

While the geography, the climate, and the lack of mountains were all irritants to me, the truth that I didn't like to admit was that I had an attitude about the people as well.

I'd been avoiding the fact that I still didn't like where I lived by focusing all of my attention on my work. My resistance was causing a problem: As long as I blamed Florida in any way, I was inhibiting my own happiness. I was going to have to learn how to like it there.

At first, that was difficult because I kept comparing Florida to Colorado, and Florida came up short every time. Just like when my motivation to lose weight was coming from comparing myself with others, comparing Florida to Colorado all the time was keeping me stuck. I realized that if I removed the comparison, I could simply find things in Florida to feel good about.

I set about deliberately searching for things to like about where I lived. While they weren't immediately apparent to me, I did find them. As I focused on those things, they gradually began to grow. Along with them, my happiness and success grew.

It wasn't always easy. I started with the smallest thing I could find to feel good about, like a flower or bird I had never seen before. As I began to collect these good feelings, I found that the more appreciation I experienced, the better I felt about this place and the more things I found to appreciate about it.

I began to notice the beauty surrounding me: Florida's ocean and rivers, wildlife, and stunning water birds. My husband and I bought a small sailboat, and we sailed on the Indian River, often with dolphins playfully darting around our boat. We watched manatees frolicking in the shallow waters and saw huge loggerhead turtles laying eggs in the sand on a gorgeous ocean beach that we could walk to from our house. We watched spectacular Kennedy Space Center shuttle launches from that same beach. I met wonderful people — right in our neighborhood — and developed close friendships.

Over time, my energy shifted. Very gradually, the things I had installed long ago, like exercise and eating well, became easier and easier because I no longer had any resistance.

I kept studying the phenomenon of personal energy and how it affects us. I learned about the principles of energy in quantum physics — that human beings are composed of energy and that our individual energy affects others.

As I continued to experience profound changes in my life, I saw the principles manifesting before my eyes. The better I felt as a result of shifting my focus toward feeling better, the better my life went. I began accomplishing goals I'd only dreamed about before.

I began to realize that I truly loved living in Florida. I felt that

I'd been given opportunities here, and a chance to make a difference, so I wanted to give back.

My husband was a volunteer fire fighter for the county, just as he had been in Colorado. Since I had met and admired the folks in his department, I applied to be on our county's Critical Incident Stress Debriefing (CISD) team.

With my counseling background, I was accepted immediately and completed their beginning through advanced training program. That gave me the special tools I needed to work with emergency service personnel who encounter tragedy in the line of duty.

It was often heart-wrenching work, but because of that training, I was able to help our police, fire, and medical teams through some of their most abrupt and dramatic events. It also helped me to better understand and guide folks through change and gave me additional tools that I still use. My involvement also gave me an even deeper appreciation for the men and women who risk their lives to help others. I'm deeply proud to have worked with them.

All of these tools became essential to my understanding of how to move through challenges. As a result of installing these practices, my life kept expanding, and it kept getting better.

Step Four:
Plan Ahead

Your body will respond to good nutrition and exercise only if you provide both regularly.

IDENTIFYING NEEDS

Do you want lots of things?

That's okay. It is natural for us to want.

Every day, we want:

- Food
- Sleep
- Clothing
- A place to sit and relax

The list goes on and on.

Needs and Feelings

You've probably noticed that as soon as you get something you wanted, you want something else. This is natural. It's not the same as greed.

Greed is the overwhelming desire to have more of something than is actually needed.

Needs are not optional. We all have them.

So what do you need?

Bodily needs—like food, water, and shelter—are basic to our survival. Personal needs are a different story. We can survive without getting our personal needs met, but they can drive our behavior or distract us when we're striving to install new intentions.

Personal needs drive our behavior because they affect our feelings. Getting your personal needs met frees you to feel good consistently, and feeling good is the key to getting the results you want.

In order to feel your best, you must:

1. Understand what your needs are
2. Design systems to get those needs met

When you identify your needs and design systems to get them met, they'll stop controlling you. You can then focus on reaching your healthy intentions. Getting your needs met allows you to move on with creating your life.

Needs List

Use the following list to identify your top ten needs, and then narrow those down to your top three. (Of course, you can also write down something that is not on the list.)

I have a need...

...to be accepted	...to direct others	...to analyze
...to be included	...for attention	...for stability
...to be encouraged	...for procedures	...to be honest
...to accomplish goals	...to be obeyed	...for luxury
...for variety	...to be noticed	...to be helped
...for checklists	...for prosperity	...for commitments
...to communicate	...to be important	...to get credit
...to help others	...to be seen	...to be praised
...to be listened to	...to be valued	...to be thanked
...to be informed	...to be accurate	...to be independent
...to keep promises	...to control	...to be useful
...to please others	...for certainty	...to be busy
...to influence others	...for recognition	...for quiet
...to be loved	...to be comfortable	...for perfection
...for consistency	...to fulfill my duties	...to be liked
...to be needed	...to have order	...to prove myself
...to follow	...for harmony	...to lead
...to have power	...to have a cause	...for responsibility
...to be respected	...for solitude	...for safety
...to perform	...to be self-reliant	...for space
...to be physically strong	...for meaningful work	

What are your top three needs?

How will you get those needs met?

UTILIZING SYSTEMS

As each minute, day, and month passes, you are either moving toward what you want or away from it. You most certainly will encounter obstacles.

- People will mistreat you.
- You will get sick.
- Things you thought were opportunities will fall through.
- Relationships will change.
- You will experience loss.

How will you keep your energy flowing in a positive direction?

How will you make good decisions when you are feeling your most vulnerable?

In order to change your life by eating better and losing weight, you'll have to plan ahead for the times when you will be tired, stressed, or scattered.

The following suggestions are developed specifically to see you through tough times or times when you are not in control of your food or of the challenges that you're facing.

Contract with Yourself

To maintain your motivation, it can help to define small, manageable targets.

1. Choose a specific action and a date by which you will complete that action.
2. Select a specific reward you'll give yourself for completing the action by that date.
3. Write down the terms in a simple contract format, and sign it.

For example:

I will go to the 8:00 a.m. exercise class this week on Monday, Wednesday, and Friday. Upon completing three exercise classes, I will reward myself with a ten-dollar bouquet of flowers.

(I eventually modified my rewards to monthly awards.)

Categorize

Your mind likes to categorize. It just makes life easier.

- Red lights mean stop
- Sharp things are dangerous

When you use this to your advantage, it can simplify your process and protect you from temptation by redefining your expectations.

When I was weaning myself off sugar, I took sweets out of the *food* category and put them in the *art* category. That way, I could appreciate beautiful desserts for the baker's artistry without eating them—because I don't eat art. I can look at art, admire it, and "ooh" and "ah" over it without eating it. By putting sweets in the same category as art, I could experience them without feeling threatened by them.

Now, I can be around desserts, and I'm okay with them. But I don't keep them in my house. I don't tempt myself with them.

I've also taken exercise out of the *recreation* category and put it in the *hygiene* category. If you think about it, most of us fussed about brushing our teeth when we were little, but then, at some point, we installed tooth brushing as a basic part of our daily hygiene. If you put exercise in the recreation category, there's an expectation that you must somehow enjoy it. Changing the category removes that expectation. After all, if you want to maintain your health, it must be a regular part of your routine, whether you enjoy it or not.

Rehearse

If you're worried about an upcoming event, simply rehearse it ahead of time.

Buffets used to scare me.

What if I couldn't control myself with all that unlimited food?

Then, I realized:

They're all basically the same. It's not like there have been a bunch of new foods invented, and I'm going to be presented with something for which I'm totally unprepared.

So I rehearsed what I would put on my plate ahead of time.

Having learned a lot about nutrition from the multitude of diet books I had read, I decided:

Okay, where might I struggle?

That would be the desserts.

Because I was a major sugar addict, I knew that the desserts would present the biggest temptation. That's when viewing them as art really helped me. This method protected me countless times.

Think about what the food choices were the last time you were at a buffet. Now, determine the healthiest choices you can make the next time, and imagine how beautiful they will look on your plate.

What will be hardest thing for you to pass up?

Re-categorize it just as I did with desserts. Most foods could be considered art, but let your imagination help you decide what works best for you.

Plan Great Evenings

Evenings are difficult for most folks because they are tired and the time is unscheduled. I used a technique that one of my clients dubbed the *Smile Jar*.

First, I repurposed business cards by writing on the back of each card one thing that I would enjoy doing in the evening.

Then, I folded the cards in half and tossed them randomly into a large-mouthed jar.

Each morning, I would reach into the jar and pick one.

Not only did this give me a specific plan for the evening; it also gave me the whole day to look forward to it (or plan further). It could be as simple as a bubble bath or a walk on the beach, but at least I'd have a plan, so that I wasn't as vulnerable during a time that was tricky for me. Using a Smile Jar added the structure I needed and prevented me from just checking out by default, like a couch potato.

Remember that you are most vulnerable when you're tired and your thoughts are scattered. This strategy can keep you focused and raise your energy during those vulnerable times.

Make Your Own Smile Jar

Write down some of the things you enjoy: things that make you smile, people you enjoy being with, and the qualities you enjoy most about those people. Use the list below to stimulate ideas.

Then, put your activity ideas in a jar, and pick one every morning to do that evening (or whenever your most difficult time is).

Use your imagination, and make it fun.

- Indoors by myself
- Indoors with others

- Outdoors by myself
- Outdoors with others
- Out and about by myself
- Out and about with others
- At work by myself
- At work with others
- Sports by myself
- Sports with others
- Reading materials
- Entertainment
- Adventures
- With my spouse
- Events
- Creative outlets
- Self-care
- Intellectual pursuits
- Volunteering

DEVELOPING NEW HABITS

All habits begin with a positive intent. The original behavior served a purpose, such as providing comfort or fulfilling a need. If the behavior satisfied your need, then you repeated it each time the need appeared.

Eventually, the behavior became a habit. As most often happens with habits, you kept doing the behavior long past its original purpose. That's how habits can become what we call *bad* or *unhealthy*, like the after-school snack.

Have you ever developed the habit of coming in the door from work, shopping, or school, and heading straight for the refrigerator?

You may not realize it or know why. You may not even eat anything. But your brain tells you that it's time for a snack.

Perhaps the habit of eating as soon as you got home served its purpose when you were growing up. After a full day of classes and activities, you were hungry. For those thirteen years, it made sense for you to come home from school every day and do the same thing.

But if you're over eighteen, you're probably not growing anymore. Maybe that habit has outlived its purpose.

Here are some guidelines for developing new habits of healthy eating and exercise. These tips provided me with the structure I needed to remove the guesswork and make the right choices for a healthy body. I hope they are helpful to you.

Shop for Food Wisely

1. SHOP THE OUTSIDE PERIMETER OF THE GROCERY STORE.

When you think about it, the real foods (i.e., those in the their natural form) are located along the outside perimeter of the grocery store. The interior aisles contain the processed food. Reroute your grocery cart to that outside perimeter, and you'll insulate yourself from the junk food until you reach the checkout counter.

2. DON'T BUY FOOD THAT CONTAINS MORE THAN THREE INGREDIENTS.

The truth is, you'd never have to worry about your weight if you ate only fresh natural food with no additives. Strive for that, but if that's not possible, at least choose foods that have very few additional ingredients. *Our bodies are designed to use foods in their natural state.*

3. BUY NOTHING AT THE CHECKOUT COUNTER.

Have you noticed that when you're standing in line at the grocery store checkout counter, there are always magazines, candy, and gum right there in your face?

Here's an idea: Find something else to look at while you're in line.

Those items are placed there to tempt a captive audience, so immunize yourself with the decision never to purchase them.

Remember: If the latest fad diet really worked, there wouldn't be a new one advertised every week.

Plan Your Eating

1. KEEP A FOOD DIARY.

Tracking your food intake is a powerful tool for gaining greater awareness of your eating patterns. Record the time, exactly what you ate, and what you were feeling at the time. (Simply recording everything you eat can help you eliminate mindless eating.)

2. "EAT BREAKFAST LIKE A KING, LUNCH LIKE A PRINCE, AND DINNER LIKE A PAUPER."

This advice from Adelle Davis served me well when I was learning how to keep weight off, and it has helped me to keep weight off all these years. If you're not used to eating breakfast, you can ease into this one, but always include protein (even if it's protein powder). This will set you up to have more energy and less hunger the rest of the day.

3. CONSIDER FIVE SMALL MEALS RATHER THAN THREE LARGE ONES.

This will distribute your food intake more evenly throughout the day. If you can't do that, then plan for a mid-morning snack and a mid-afternoon snack. Keep your body well fueled throughout the day, and you'll be much less likely to grab a snack that you'll end up regretting.

Healthy snack ideas can include:

- High-protein, low-sugar nutrition bar
- Apples or celery with peanut or almond butter
- Baggies of cut up raw vegetables and fruit
- Blended green drink (fresh vegetables, water, protein powder, banana, and ice)
- Six almonds (or a small portion of another healthy protein)
- Four Medjool dates (pricey, but deliciously sweet and indulgent)
- Unsweetened whole-grain cereal

4. NEVER LEAVE THE HOUSE WITHOUT YOUR COOLER PACKED.

This will make it easier for you to stick to your healthy eating routine. Don't allow yourself to be at the mercy of fast food restaurants. Find some healthy snacks that you enjoy eating, and then pack a small personal cooler with those foods every day.

Note: Make sure you include protein. Fruits and veggies are great, of course, but combine them with protein, and you'll stay satisfied much longer.

5. USE A SMALLER PLATE.

Research has shown that people who used a ten-inch plate rather than a twelve-inch plate ate 22 percent fewer calories. If you're used to eating huge portions, this can help you naturally scale your portions down.

6. ELIMINATE ALL FLAVORED BEVERAGES.

Because most of us need to be drinking more water than we do (not to mention less sugar, caffeine, and additives), it's best to limit our daily beverage choices to water. Even self-proclaimed *diet* or *zero-calorie* sodas contain additives and carbonation.

Neither is good for you, so begin to eliminate any reliance on them.

7. GET CREATIVE WITH HERBS AND SPICES.

As you eat more natural whole foods, you'll be retraining your taste buds. If you're used to eating lots of sugar, fat, and processed foods, this new way of eating may seem very bland. That's because you've been artificially stimulating your palate.

Bridge the gap with fresh herbs (which you can easily grow on a window sill) and spices, or add a little liquid aminos (found in most grocery or natural foods stores). Soon, your taste buds will adjust, and fresh foods will taste good.

8. SAVOR MEALTIME.

Never eat on the run. Slow the pace of your eating. Take smaller bites, and savor your food. Stop eating when you feel satisfied rather than full (go for 80 percent full). Once you feel satisfied, shift your focus to family members or an enjoyable task.

9. LIMIT (OR ELIMINATE) ALCOHOL.

Basically, alcohol turns to sugar in your body, so it's best to put it in the treat category. Some folks find that a small glass of wine every day doesn't inhibit their weight loss. It may, however, relax your resolve. Just beware, and don't let the occasional indulgence throw off your healthy eating pattern.

Since alcohol has no nutritional value, at best, you're ingesting calories without feeding your body, and at worst, it could be leaching vitamins from your body and dehydrating you.

10. MAKE FRUIT YOUR DESSERT IF YOU MUST HAVE SOMETHING SWEET.

If you're in the habit of having a sweet after meals, substitute fresh or dried fruit (a few dates may suffice). This should eliminate any craving, but be sure to shift your focus too. Push yourself away from the table, and go for a walk.

11. DON'T EAT WITHIN THREE HOURS OF BEDTIME.

Depending on your schedule, this may be difficult. Just remember that eating lots of food right before you go to sleep will add weight to your body. It's best to have at least two hours without food before retiring for the night.

Ideally, you would have a light dinner, followed by some light physical activity (like a short walk, some stretching, or a ping-pong game), followed by a routine to help you wind down, like hot chamomile tea and a half hour of pleasure reading before bed.

12. USE THE TWENTY MINUTE RULE.

It takes about twenty minutes for your body to realize that you ate, so slowing down or delaying helps. (My inner robot would have me wolfing down food faster than my body could register that I had eaten. Then in twenty minutes, I'd be sick.)

To help you slow down and be mindful of your body's responses, eat a moderate amount of healthy food, and then, stop and set a timer for twenty minutes. Leave the table, the kitchen, and any other eating cues behind, and focus on something else for twenty minutes. Then, ask yourself if you're still hungry. You may find that you've forgotten all about eating.

13. REMEMBER: YOU ARE WHAT YOU EAT.

If you want to look and feel healthy, you must feed your body what it needs and eliminate what damages it. A steady flow of nutrients, water, and oxygen—along with plenty of exercise—helps your organs (including your brain) function properly and will help your circulatory system support your vital organs. *Good looks and good health depend on good nutrition and exercise.* There's no way around that.

Foods to focus on:

- Vegetables
- Fruits
- Whole grains
- Healthy proteins

Things to avoid:

- Sugars (including fructose and high-fructose corn syrup)
- Trans fats
- Saturated fats
- Refined, enriched, or bleached flours

14. WHEN IN DOUBT, DRINK WATER.

If you find yourself rummaging around for food when you're actually bored, tired, or just plain out of sorts, drink a large glass of water instead. That distractibility you're feeling may simply be dehydration. Your brain cannot store water and must be rehydrated often in order to function at its best. (Ideally, two to four ounces every half hour.)

Often, when we're easily distracted or feeling out of sorts, we're actually dehydrated. Just remember that your body benefits from drinking water, and at the very least, it won't do you any harm.

15. BE AWARE OF EATING CUES.

You may not realize it, but even subtle things like what you're wearing or where you're sitting can influence eating behavior. To stay alert, change your patterns. Never change into *eating clothes* when you are at home. (You know the ones: loose-fitting caftans or baggy sweatpants that make you completely unaware of your body.) Instead, change into workout clothes that help you want to move.

Plan Your Exercise

1. GET A WORKOUT BUDDY.

Having a supportive partner to be accountable to can help a great deal on this journey. Just make sure you choose someone who is as committed as you are. And don't hesitate to enlist the advice of qualified nutritionists and personal trainers along the way. You can't have too much support when you're installing healthy habits.

2. TRY A CLASS.

The nice thing about a class is that it happens at a specific time, which forces you to build it into your schedule. I have found that attending classes helps me maintain the discipline to show up at the gym at a certain time *and* exercise for the full class (rather than wimping out after ten minutes on my own). If you're intimidated by a class full of people, just remember that they were all beginners at one point, and they all remember what that's like, so they're on your side.

3. CONSIDER EARLY MORNING EXERCISE.

Exercise takes dedicated time, so make sure you give it a place in your schedule that you won't be tempted to reprioritize at the last minute. You may find that early morning is the only time you can absolutely guarantee that you'll be be able to exercise, uninterrupted, regularly. (Personally, I found that too many things came up to pull me off track if I waited until later in the day.)

Experiment with best times for you, but don't let *I'm not a morning person* be your excuse. Your body can be trained to wake up earlier. (If I can train myself, anybody can!)

4. MAKE AN ABSOLUTE COMMITMENT TO EXERCISING THREE TO FOUR TIMES PER WEEK.

If you think about it, anything new that you undertake is always hardest at the beginning. Exercise is no different. Learning new movements takes concentration, so your mind may feel fatigued. Your muscles will probably be sore as they adjust to the added demands.

If you allow yourself to rest for too long, you'll be starting over all the time. That's frustrating, not to mention, hard on your body.

Movement helps alleviate the pain of sore muscles by moving lactic acid out of your body. If you're sore, *move.* Your muscles will adapt and reward you with greater strength and more stamina. Stick with it for a minimum of three months, and if you get bored, then change your routine. Don't be afraid to try new things.

5. LIMIT NON-EXERCISE DAYS TO THREE.

Set a boundary with yourself that you will never go more than three days without exercising. If you allow yourself to be sedentary for too long following strenuous exercise, you'll deprive yourself of the benefits of all that hard work. Your body will respond to good nutrition and exercise only if you provide both regularly.

Chapter Five

A New Perspective

I was never more grateful that I had installed healthy habits than when I began to lose my family members.

First, my parents, who had lived in Colorado, also moved to Florida because my brother—who had gotten married and lived in Atlanta—had a child. He was their first grandchild, and they wanted to be closer, so they moved halfway between my brother and me.

When this grandchild was only two years old, my brother became ill and was hospitalized. His heart stopped, he was on life support for six weeks, and then, he died. That profound event rocked my boat, but I used my knowledge of the Change Cycle to feel the things I needed to feel in order to move through it.

At that point, my mother kind of unhooked, and her health began to decline. Four years later, she passed away, and four years after that, my dad passed away.

In a period of about eight years, I had lost them all.

Thinking that there must have been a reason why I was still alive, I reexamined everything about my life, recommitted to it in a very new way, and sought more tools to help myself feel better and stay on track. While I had found work that I truly loved, I was with the right person, I was where I was supposed to be, and I was doing what I had a calling to do, I felt totally unprepared for these losses.

As I moved through the grief and tried to focus on all the blessings I had with my family, I vowed to keep myself healthy – *for them*. This was especially important for me as I was going through this transition, and it reminded me of something that I had learned about years earlier in my efforts to become a better counselor – a concept developed in the early twentieth century by Jewish philosopher and educator, Martin Buber, called *I-Thou and I-It*. While I didn't recall it making much of an impression back then, now that I knew something about quantum physics, it suddenly made perfect sense to me.

According to Buber's philosophy, because humans are composed of energy, they respond to the energy of other humans. In other words, human energy can be felt by other humans. When you regard another human being as a fellow person (I-Thou), it can be felt. In the same way, when you regard another human being not as a fellow person but as an object (I-It), that can also be felt. Because human beings respond according to how they feel, and because in physics, like energy attracts like energy, human beings will match their energy with how they feel they are being regarded.

I learned that:

- Human energy interacts with the energy of others.
- This interaction of energy is what creates the results that happen in our lives.
- Everything in life happens because our lives are created with others.

That was a huge revelation to me.

While it was true that, for the first time in my life, I had been feeling very proud that I was good at something, my reasons to keep myself healthy and fit had really been for me. Yes, I did want to be better for my clients, but being good at something had been a point of pride for me.

Now, I understood that whether I liked it or not, my life was being created with other people. As much as I wanted to give myself full credit, the truth of the matter was that results are really co-created.

Once I got that through my head, I knew that I needed to pay attention. My learning opened up a whole new way for me to think about my physical body and just how I affected others. It led me to examine a lot of my attitudes, and I began to rely less and less on my work for my identity. This was very important because, frankly, I had become overly work-focused even though I had a lot to be grateful for in my personal life.

Dieting is a very self-focused activity. When I was struggling with my weight, I didn't want other people to know that I was eating a whole bag of candy, so I would isolate myself. (That's classic addictive behavior, by the way.) Then, when I felt bad about myself for overeating, I wasn't very nice to people (if I engaged with them at all, which was rare).

Now that I had installed practices to protect my health and keep me feeling good physically — and was continually learning tools to cope with all the loss and grief — I was feeling better emotionally. The better I felt about myself, the better I was for others.

Step Five:
Co-Create Your Life

When your focus becomes much larger than just you...

When you truly embrace living with others...

When you make choices based on what will help you be your best for them...

... then, the struggle finally ends, and a new life begins.

UNDERSTANDING INTERACTIONS

There is an invisible component that lies beneath your behavior and affects your outcomes, and it is critical to your success.

This essential component is your *way of being* toward others.

Your way of being is an energy that can be felt, and it has an impact on the people around you. The same event or action can have completely different outcomes depending on your intention and the choices you make relative to others.

Seeing Others as Objects

In every interaction, you have two choices:

1. To see the other as a person
2. To see the other as an object

When you see someone as a person:

- You recognize that they are real, just like you, and have cares and concerns that they are dealing with too.

As a result:

- You are able to respond to their needs and to invite and inspire their best, which leads to increased trust and creates results.

When you see someone as an object:

- You view them as something that's in your way (an obstacle), something that you can use (a vehicle), or something that's insignificant (irrelevant).

As a result:

- You begin to justify yourself and blame them, which provokes negativity and creates *collusion*.

Collusion is the understood cooperation between people to do something underhanded. It's a good word here because of the unspoken agreement that it implies. ***When you treat someone as an object, they treat you as an object.*** That's how the collusion takes place. This cycle leads to an inability to focus on results.

The best way to illustrate this is with an example.

Here's the situation:

You have made an intention to lose weight. You have shared this with your husband, children, and coworkers. It's day three, and you have just come home from work. It's your husband's turn to prepare dinner. He shows up with takeout from your favorite Italian restaurant. He bought your usual chicken Parmesan dinner.

Here are two possible responses:

1. *My husband has been at work today too. He was probably too tired to cook dinner, or he could have been unprepared or just out of ideas.*

- It doesn't matter why he didn't cook. The fact is that he brought home chicken Parmesan for you. You scrape off the breading and cheese, eat the chicken, leave the pasta, eat the salad, and then, go for a walk.

2. *My husband is sabotaging me. I make him healthy dinners all the time, but when he's supposed to get dinner, he doesn't consider what I need.*

- You don't want to fight, so you eat all of your Italian dinner (*after all, it was paid for*) and watch television. The next day, you feel bloated and resentful and struggle to get back to eating healthy.

Which response do you think will make the most impact and create a different result from your husband the next time it's his turn to cook dinner?

Can you see how your choice, your intent to treat him as a person just like you, and your intent to be healthy can create the results you want?

I know this is a simple example, but sometimes things will go wrong. You do *not* have to move away from what you want when that happens. Those are simply obstacles that you have to overcome. *Your way of being with others will make those obstacles disappear when you treat others as people just like you.*

Seeing Yourself and Others as People

In order to invite better responses, you must eliminate the labels you have given yourself and others. You can change your perception of them *and* of yourself. When you change how you regard yourself and others, the energy shifts and opens the door for others to match your energy.

When you see yourself as a problem to be solved, you'll continually create problems. That's an energy match. It's not your fault. You don't realize what you're attracting.

You begin to see yourself as:

- Irrelevant
- Inferior
- An obstacle
- Unimportant

When you do this, your heart is at war.

When you see yourself and others as a people, you'll understand that you are all equal in all ways.

You see that their…

- Hopes
- Needs
- Cares
- Fears

…are as real and important as your own.

When you do this, your heart is at peace.

Figure 11. People or Objects

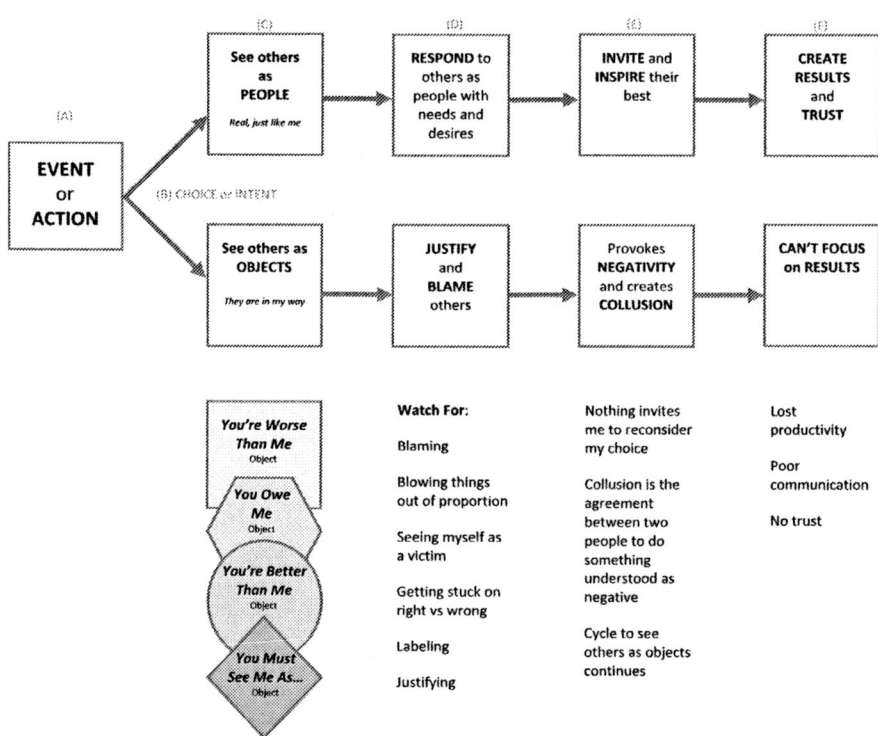

In Figure 12, the Life Principles Spring Coil (Figure 6, page X) has been changed slightly to show how your way of being defines your outcomes. The arrow shooting through the coil represents your way of being. As much as you might like to think that you're in this life alone, your experiences are created in conjunction with others.

Figure 12. Creating New Results

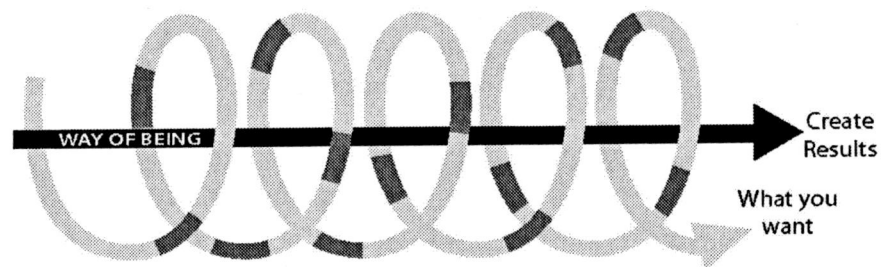

Keep in mind that each dark spot represents a thought. Events happen before your thoughts. Immediately after an event, you think. What you think is based on what you believe about that event, and what you believe is based on previous repeated thoughts and outcomes.

Remember, you either move forward or backward around the coil. When you make a deliberate choice to focus on what you want, you will increase your energy and get a positive outcome. When you do that you create results and get what you want. With practice, you can perfect this and you will accomplish more than you ever imagined.

Keeping Your Focus on What You Can Control

Virtually every situation in your life can be divided into three parts:

1. What YOU bring to the situation, such as:

    • Your personality
    • Your family history
    • Your mood
    • Your hopes and dreams

2. The FACTS about the situation:

    • Just what is so
    • With no emotions
    • As if a reporter were covering it

3. What OTHERS bring to the situation, such as:

    • Their personalities
    • Their family histories
    • Their moods
    • Their hopes and dreams

The bad news is that you have no control over the FACTS box or the OTHERS box.

None.

Zip.

The good news is that you have *total control* of your own box.

Figure 13. The Box You Control

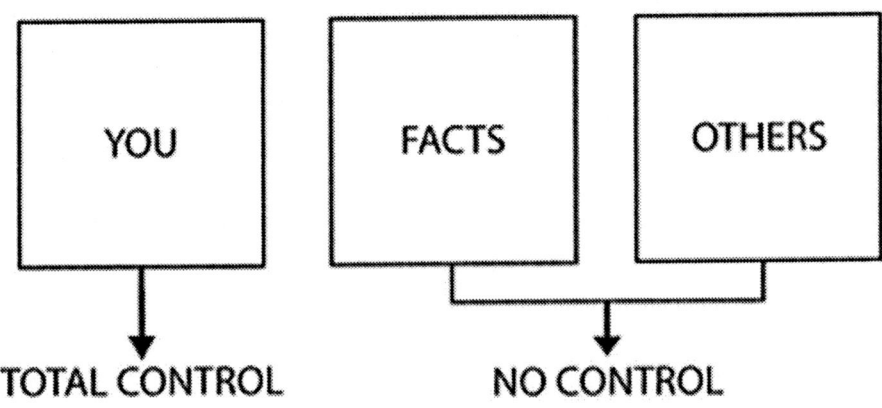

When you worry about or try to change things outside your control, you'll feel bad because you have no control in those boxes. (If you've ever tried to change another person, you know exactly what I mean.)

When you focus your attention upon what is within your control, you access your creative power.

Focus on your own box, for that is where true change begins.

When I first learned this, it really set me free. Without realizing it, I had been spending a lot of time working those other boxes, thinking that if I could just get them all lined up, then I would feel good. But even when it had seemed like that was working, the result had always been short-lived.

Typically, at any moment in time, the only thing in your box is a feeling. If you take full responsibility for that feeling, you can usually make it better.

When I've shared this concept with kids, they totally get it. They understand that working the other boxes squanders your energy. If you're going to create change in your life, you need energy, so don't squander it on things over which you have no control.

This understanding has helped me a lot. I encourage you to use it to keep you focused as you move through the process of creating change in your life.

LIMITING TOXIC EXPOSURE

Sometimes, there are people in your environment who are detrimental to you. While it may sound harsh, the best thing you can do is to consider them toxic and limit your exposure to them. Setting clear boundaries with these people, confronting them, or just learning to deal with their anger will allow you to protect yourself.

The following tools can help you to deal with these situations, so you can focus on what you want.

Setting Clear Boundaries

Setting boundaries is simply a way of educating others about what is important to you. Your boundaries are the defined limits that you communicate regarding the behavior of others. Keep in mind that others cannot know where your boundaries are unless you tell them.

1. Begin with a value statement:

- "I care about our relationship, so I want to clarify something."
- "I'm sure it's not intentional, but I must ask you to..."
- "We're on the same team, so I need to let you know something."

2. Define the boundary:

- "I need..."
- "I prefer to be called..."
- "I don't allow anyone to..."
- "It's not acceptable to me for anyone to..."
- "I'd appreciate it if you would..."

3. Explain why it's important to you:

- "This is why..."
- "I guess it's because..."
- "It makes me feel..."
- "It's just a quirk I have."

4. End with a question, to check for understanding and agreement:

- "Okay?"
- "Can you understand where I'm coming from?"
- "Would you be willing to...?"
- "What would you be willing to do?"

Confrontation

For many people, confrontation is avoided at all costs. I'm sure you know others who seem to seek confrontation. In either case, we all have to deal with conflict or disagreements at some point.

Here's a method you can use to support you in this process:

1. Think through (ahead of time) what you want to say.
2. Speak in a *neutral* but firm tone, and don't get emotional.

"When you _____ (behavior or verbal communication), it causes a problem because _____ (reason). In the future, I ask that you _____ (positive action). Do you understand?"

   3. *Stop talking,* and wait for an answer.

Dealing with Angry People

Angry people can be the biggest energy drain of all. These people are out of your control, and many times, they are not thinking clearly. ***The best way to deal with anger is to diffuse it.***

Anger comes from being:

- Scared
- Confused
- Frustrated

Often, people just want to know that they have been heard and that what they are saying matters. Let the person get it all out, and wait to respond until it's clear that they are finished or until they ask for a response.

Try these short phrases, and then, *stop talking.*

SIMPLE RESPONSE: "I appreciate you bringing that to my attention."

FULL AGREEMENT: "You're right." or "Yes."

PARTIAL AGREEMENT: "You may be right."

VALIDATE: "You have a point."

HUMOR (*not* sarcasm): "I guess I dropped the ball on that one!"

REFLECT FEELINGS: "Sounds like you're really upset with me."

DEFLECT: "I'm trying something new."

SHIFT GEARS: "Could we talk in fifteen minutes?"

BEING YOUR BEST FOR OTHERS

Success happens through focus and feeling good. You don't get there by trying to make it easier; you get there by making yourself better.

Examining Your Intentions

If you desire different outcomes in your life, always begin by examining your intentions.

Are they inclusive of others and your environment?

Be in a continuous learning mode. Remember that the outcome created in any given situation is the result of your energy in combination with the energy of others and the environment.

In other words:

- Your intention
- What you invite from others
- What you invite from the environment

...all work together to produce your results.

Considering Your Context

Keep in mind that life is in relationship with others. If you have a problem with weight, while it may seem like *your* problem and only yours, like all problems, you have it among other people. If you are going to lose weight or maintain your weight, it's true that you're the one who must begin to do it.

In that respect, it is about you.

But it may be useful to wonder what has kept you from doing it in the past. You have to keep in mind that nothing is *just* about you. While you may be the one who has a desire to lose weight, you do that in the context of your life with others.

When you begin to realize…

- That *everything* you experience happens in the context of your life with others
- That others, in fact, have hopes, dreams, and concerns just like you

…then you can understand that your desire to lose weight also involves your attitude toward others.

You might be motivated to do — or *not* do — something because of certain ways you're seeing others or certain ways that you're justifying how you're seeing yourself.

When you recognize that your life occurs with others, and you become more open and engage with others more, then you're far less likely to isolate yourself and do any of the damaging things you might do if you were only focused on yourself.

The bottom line is: ***When you become aware that what you do affects others, you make better choices.***

Reevaluating Your *Why*

When you notice that you are focusing only on yourself or eating in a way that makes you feel bad, ask yourself:

Do I withdraw from other people?

Does that help me to be my best around others, or does it make me want to retreat?

Does it make me less than what I would like to be around others?

If you change *why* you lose weight, maintain weight, or keep yourself healthy, and you start doing it for others, then everything changes.

- It provides broader reasons for your selections and behaviors.
- Changing becomes easier.
- It limits self-focus, the very thing that has kept you stuck.

When your focus becomes much larger than just you...

When you truly embrace living with others...

When you make choices based on what will help you be your best for them...

...then, the struggle finally ends, and a new life begins.

Conclusion

As I stated at the beginning of the book, this process is very simple, but it's not easy. It takes practice and the right tools to get results.

It does not take willpower.

There is no such thing as a willpower muscle.

You can let go of that myth.

Sometimes, the biggest error in our thinking is that we focus on what we don't want. When you say that you want to lose weight, it may feel like you are focusing on what you want, but in reality, that's focusing on what you *don't* want.

When things are tough…

When nothing is going right…

When problems seem to keep popping up out of nowhere…

…you are *resisting* what is.

You're out of your box, and it's time to stop and examine where your focus lies.

Resistance creates more of what you don't want. When you make the deliberate choice to direct your energy toward what you *do* want, you'll feel resistance disappear.

Partner with your subconscious. Don't ignore it. Use it to your favor by letting it help you. There will be a period of time during which you might feel like it's pulling you back. It just doesn't want you to be disappointed, that's all.

Eventually, though, those voices will calm down. I can promise you that because I have experienced the change in my own subconscious. Those voices have calmed within me, and they actually encourage me now.

Remember:

1. Repeated thoughts become beliefs.
2. Beliefs drive behaviors.
3. Repeated behaviors become habits.

The life that you create basically boils down to your habits, your beliefs, and your moment-to-moment focus, so pay attention to how you feel because that will tell you what you're focused on. Find positive things to feel good about, and you can succeed with anything that you try.

I wasn't making any progress at all until I started focusing on how much I wanted those jeans with the pockets close together. That was the first time I had even one bead on what I actually wanted. I didn't have a clue about what it would take for that to happen. I didn't know what my weight would have to be, what size those pants would be, or anything else. I just had this image—at eighteen years old—of what it would be like to wear them.

As I moved forward, my reasons evolved.

The biggest change and the thing that helped me the most was to make my reason be about others.

Remember:

*   I got out of the window and didn't kill myself because it would hurt my parents. That became a compelling reason. It was about something beyond me.
*   I recommitted to exercise because I realized that I became a better counselor when I felt better. It made me more mentally alert. That was about being better for others.
*   I vowed to keep myself healthy to honor the memory of my family and to ensure that I would be here for my nephew.

That's a huge component. If you want to change your physical body, try making the change for others. It can keep you moving through the change cycles much more efficiently.

When you are in doubt about your direction or what to do next, consider the following:

Choose Positive Self-Talk

- Reach for better-feeling thoughts
- Reframe situations
- Visualize positive outcomes
- Amplify the benefits

Remove Energy Drains...

...in your thinking.
...in your actions.
...in your environment.

Make Amends and Forgive Others

Forgiving others helps us forgive ourselves and make peace with the past.

Utilize Obstacles

Obstacles are necessary. Overcoming them changes you forever.

Ask yourself:

- *What's good about this?*
- *Is it in my box?*

Instead of Stewing, Shift to Problem Solving

- If you can't shift in one minute, change the subject.
- Don't work at it, play with it.
- Just imagine it, relax enough to let it happen, and it *will* happen.

Don't feed your mind junk food.

That's the worst thing, and it leads to other unhealthy things.

You can keep yourself in a healthy cycle by watching how you think and practicing positive thoughts. While you can't monitor your thoughts all day long, you can start by paying attention to how you feel. That will let you know what you're focused on. The most important thing is that you feel good because then, you have trained your mind to focus on what you want rather than what you don't want.

If you end up feeling bad or notice a drop in your energy, reach for thoughts that help you feel better. Have a handful of thoughts that reliably help you feel better, and you'll get your energy back. It's all about refocusing.

Your next thought will either raise your energy or lower it; the choice is yours.

When you remove the noise of negative thinking habits and consistently practice focusing upon what you want, mental disturbances will lessen, and you'll allow new beliefs to take root.

As your thinking becomes more positively focused:

- Your actions will follow more easily.
- You'll be more decisive and better able to align your actions with your newly-formed beliefs.
- Your energy will increase.
- You will be able to manifest what you want.
- Life will become simpler.

Results are much more than an achievement; they are the state of being that you have reached.

By being in the present, you will learn how to enjoy your life. You'll create clear intentions, continue expanding your awareness, and direct your own energy. And along the way, your intentions will begin to come true.

This process has no end, and the parts are interwoven.

With increased awareness and practice, your intentions will begin to show up in your life. Over time, you will likely find yourself surpassing what you originally thought was possible. You will be able to make conscious decisions about your life as it is happening, and you'll feel confident about your life choices. As you practice directing your energy, you'll find it affecting every area of your life. This will create positive change in many areas, which will reinforce your motivation to continue.

This is the route to creating a fulfilling life. If a shorter path existed, I would have found it!

About the Author

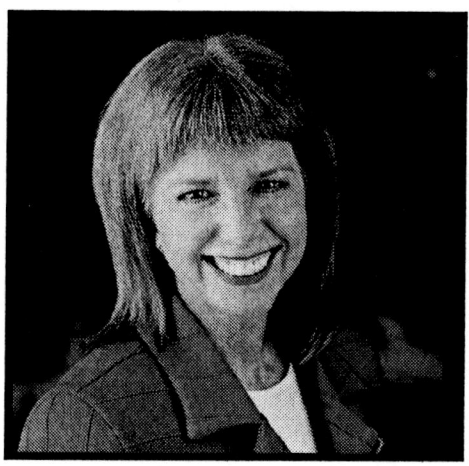

Linda K. Cobb is dedicated to helping people lead their best lives. Raised by a heart-centered hospital president, she witnessed the powerful impact that one person can make within an organization, a community, or a family. That role model sparked her desire to find proven tools to help leaders of all kinds create a positive impact. Believing that today's world requires us all to be leaders of our own lives, she continuously seeks out the best tools to help that happen.

Linda is a coach, speaker, author, and trainer with over twenty-five years of experience. Having personally coached hundreds of leaders and trained thousands in her life-changing programs, she is passionate about human potential and wellness, and she advocates updating coping strategies to reflect life's ever-evolving circumstances. As owner/president of The Coaching Company, Inc. since 1997, Linda is dedicated to life and leadership coaching. Her proven processes for coaching, behavior change, and facilitation have been widely used, both locally and nationally. Her clients are those seeking personal or professional development and life satisfaction.

Linda has a Master of Science degree in personnel psychology and is a graduate of Coach University and the Arbinger Institute's *Mastery in Coaching and Facilitating* program. She holds certifications in neurolinguistic programming (NLP), corporate coaching, retirement coaching, and advanced trauma debriefing as well as numerous assessments.

Coach Cobb is also the author of *Directions: A Guide for Life*, a flip book of key principles and strategies to help leaders create results most efficiently, as well as *The Thrive Guide for Caregivers*, a book of practical tools to help family caregivers maintain their sanity, relationships, and health.

Linda's philosophy is:

Love large. Travel light.

"*Love large* shifts my focus to offering my greatest value to others in the largest way I can. That eliminates the isolation of self-focus and restores energy. *Travel light* helps me maintain a light attitude through life's many changes and reminds me that by fully accessing the remarkable resources of my mind, body, and spirit, I always have everything I need."

She believes:

"Coaching is ideal for busy people who want to be more successful because it's action-oriented, convenient, and focused on creating a future by design rather than by default."

Linda's unique approach has been successfully utilized for leadership development, management training, weight-management programs, and life-transition coaching.

Learn more about her at:

www.lindacobb.com